PROFESSIONAL SERVICES FOR MEN:

HAIRCUTTING AND ST

THOMSON
DELMAR LEARNING

Australia   Canada   Mexico   Singapore   Spain   United Kingdom   Unite

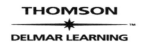

Milady's Professional Services for Men: Haircutting and Styling

President, Milady:
Dawn Gerrain

Director of Learning Solutions:
Sherry Dickinson

Acquisitions Editor:
Brad Hanson

Product Manager:
Erik Herman

Editorial Assistant:
Jessica Burns

Director of Content and Media Productions:
Wendy A. Troeger

Content Project Manager:
Nina Tucciarelli

Associate Content Project Manager:
Angela Iula

Composition:
Carlisle Publishing Services

Director of Marketing:
Wendy Mapstone

Marketing Channel Manager:
Sandra Bruce

Marketing Coordinator:
Nicole Riggi

Cover Design:
Essence of Seven

Library of Congress Cataloging-in-Publication Data:
Milady's professional services for men : haircutting and styling.
     p. cm. — (Professional services for men)
  Includes index.
  ISBN-10: 1-4180-5089-X
  ISBN-13: 978-1-4018-8169-6
  1. Haircutting. 2. Hairdressing. I. Milady Publishing Company. II. Title: Hair cutting and styling. III. Series.
  TT960.M56 2006
  646.7'24—dc22

                         2006016060

NOTICE TO THE READER

TABLE OF CONTENTS

PREFACE

A resurgence of barbers, barbershops, and barbering is taking place nationwide as the male consumer once again seeks the ambience and services of a real barbershop. To meet the growing needs and demands of their male clientele, many shops are finding they must offer a full range of professional hair and skin care services for men—it is no longer enough to offer just a good cut. Have you found yourself in this position? Are you an experienced barber who needs to learn more about male skin care and facial hair design? Or are you interested in managing your own shop? Do you know all there is to know about cutting and styling but find hair coloring or hair restoration a new challenge to you? Do you want to add men's services to your salon or day spa and need information specific to caring for male clientele? Or, are you new to the profession and want to learn about the fundamentals of cutting and styling, or seek a barbering position? Whatever the case may be, the *Professional Services for Men* series is for you.

Thomson Delmar Learning has created a series of concise, informative books designed to help professional barbers and stylists develop the skills necessary to meet the growing needs of their male clientele. The four books in the series are:

Professional Services for Men: Facial Massage, Shaving, and Hair Design

Professional Services for Men: Haircoloring and Hair Restoration

Professional Services for Men: Haircutting and Styling

Professional Services for Men: Career Management for Barbers

Each book presents the need-to-know information in an easy to understand format. Utilizing numerous full-color images and drawings, straightforward language, and helpful features such as "Tech Terms," "FYI," "Caution," and "Focus On," for added learning enrichment in your profession. To enhance your learning, the first three books take you step-by-step through the fundamental techniques of hair and skin care for men while emphasizing client comfort and safety. The last book in the *Professional Services for Men* series moves away from the technical aspects of providing men's services and looks toward the career management side of the profession.

In this, the third book in the series, the fundamentals of haircutting and styling are explained. Beginning with a review of the client consultation and moving through the principles and techniques of cutting and styling, *Professional Services for Men: Haircutting and Styling* is a comprehensive overview of what you will need to know to provide the hair care services your male clientele seek. Specifically, you will learn about *facial shapes* and *head forms* so you can achieve consistent and successful haircutting results. You will review key *haircutting terminology* so you and other barbers and stylists will be speaking the same language. You will walk step-by-step through numerous haircutting techniques such as the *fingers-and-shear technique, shear-over-comb technique,* and *arching technique,* as well as *clipper cutting, razor cut-*

ting, and *outline shaving.* Finally, you will receive an introduction to hairstyling. In it, you will learn the basics of *blow-dry styling* and *finger waving,* as well as techniques for styling hair into *braids* and *locks.*

So, whether haircutting and styling are new to you, or you are just looking for a refresher, you will find what you are looking for in this exciting and informative book!

A very special thank you to the following individuals for their contributions and assistance with the Professional Men's Services series:

Maura T. Scali-Sheahan, Master Barber and Educator
Cory Cole, Master Barber
Laura Downs, Barber
Greg Zorian, Jr., Master Barber
Greg Zorian, III, Master Barber
Helen Wos, Instructor/Barber
Lorilee Bird, Student Barber
Mark Blue, Student Barber
Christopher Morris, Student Barber
Kristen Santa Lucia, Student Barber

Andis, William Marvy Company, Wahl, and 44/20 for use of their product photographs.

Gregory's Barbershop, Clifton Park, NY for use of their location.

Morris Flamingo, Inc. for use of the Campbell Lather King.

Photography Credits:

Section opener photo, Figures 36–46, 48–54, 60–62, 64–68, 70–93, 95–101, 103–106, 133–137, 147–195, 198a–248, 252–269, 271–277, Paul Castle Photography
Figure 69, courtesy of Morris Flamingo, Inc.
Figures 94 and 107, courtesy of Anetta Nadolna
Figures 249–251, 270, photographed by Preston Phillips for Milady's "The Multicultural Client"

PROFESSIONAL SERVICES FOR MEN:
HAIRCUTTING AND STYLING

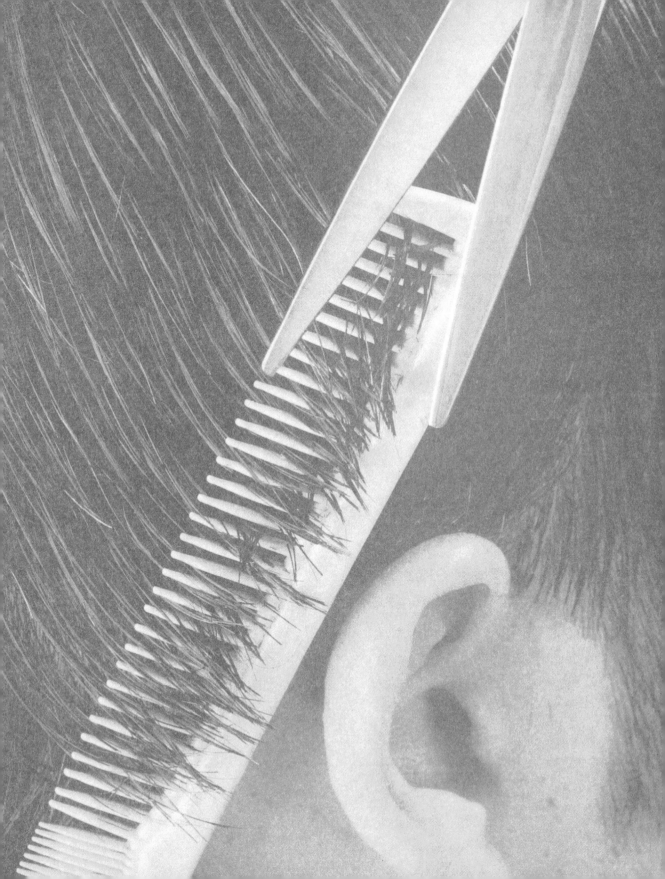

HAIRCUTTING AND STYLING

1

The art of haircutting involves individualized and precise designing, cutting, and shaping of the hair. In order to perform the art of haircutting successfully, the barber must be at ease using a variety of tools, implements, techniques, and methods.

It is important to remember that a good haircut is the foundation of a good hairstyle. To achieve optimal results requires knowning the proper way to cut, blend, and taper the hair using clippers, shears, and razors. Practice and application are necessary for the achievement and refinement of these skills because each new client will present new challenges and learning opportunities that form the basis for future success.

The hairstyle, and therefore the haircut, should accentuate the client's strong features and minimize the weaker ones. The client's head shape, facial contour, neckline, and hair texture must be taken into consideration. The barber needs to be guided by the client's wishes, personality, and lifestyle as well.

THE CLIENT CONSULTATION

A thorough client consultation helps to eliminate any guesswork about the haircut or style to be performed. This is the time when the barber must determine just what it is the client is asking for in the way of a haircut or style. Phrases such as "a little off the top" or "over the ears" are not specific enough for haircutting purposes. How is "a little" measured? Is it 1/4 inch or 1 inch? Does "over-the-ears" mean covering the ears or cutting around the ears? These interpretations are just two examples of why the consultation is so important to both the client and the barber.

Some basic questions that barbers should ask the client before the actual cutting begins are as follows:

- How long has it been since your last haircut?

  Knowing that the average hair growth is about 1/2 inch per month allows the barber to envision the preferred length of the hair before it grew out and needed to be cut again.

- Do you prefer a similar style or are you looking for something new?

  The answer to this question can lead the barber directly to the cutting stage or to further discussion with the client about appropriate styles and options.

- What is your usual morning routine (shampoo, blow-dry, etc.)?

  The answer will indicate how much time the client is willing to spend on hair care.

- Are you having any particular problems with your hairstyle?

- This question provides an opportunity to open dialogue about specific hair-related issues such as problem areas, length, fullness, growth and wave patterns, hair texture, density, or color.

Additional consultation questions should lead to answers that help the barber to determine the length of the sideburns, the shape of the neckline, and whether or not the client desires a neck shave, eyebrow trim, and so on. With practice and experience, barbers learn the questions to ask.

Envisioning is the process of picturing or visualizing in your mind the finished cut and style based on what the client has told you. With the information gained through the consultation, the barber is better able to visualize the client's expectations of the haircutting service. It is essential to achieve this understanding *before* beginning the haircut.

BASIC PRINCIPLES OF HAIRCUTTING AND STYLING

Each haircut is a representation and advertisement of the barber's work. Remember, a good haircut is the foundation of a good hairstyle.

Hairstyling has been defined as the artistic cutting and dressing of hair to best fit the client's physical needs and personality. Pay attention to details such as client comfort, sideburn lengths, outlines, balance, and proportion. The consultation should provide sufficient information about the client's lifestyle and personality to suggest a suitable style, but a study of facial shapes assists the barber in determining the *best* style for a client's features.

Facial Shapes

The facial shape of each individual is determined by the position and prominence of the facial bones. There are seven general facial shapes: oval, round, inverted triangular, square, pear-shaped, oblong, and diamond. In order to recognize each facial shape and then be able to give correct advice, the barber should be acquainted with the outstanding characteristics of each type. With this information, the barber can suggest a haircut and style that complements the facial shape in much the same way certain clothes flatter the body.

The following facial shapes should constitute a guide for choosing an appropriate style:

■ *Oval:* The oval-shaped face is generally recognized as the ideal shape. Any hairstyle that maintains the oval shape is usually suitable (Figure 1). Try changing the

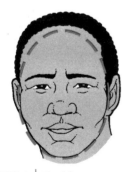

FIGURE 1 | Oval face.

part. Experiment, but keep in mind elements such as the client's lifestyle, comfort, and ease of maintenance.

- *Round:* The aim here is to slim the face. Hair that is too short will emphasize fullness, so create some height on the top to lengthen the look of the face (Figure 2). An off-center part and some waves at eye level will also help lessen the full appearance of the face. Beards should be styled to make the face appear oval.

- *Inverted triangular:* The potential problems with this facial shape are overwide cheekbones and a narrow jaw line (Figure 3). Keep the hair close at the crown and temples and longer in back, or try changing the part and the direction of the hair. A full beard helps to fill out the narrow jaw.

- *Square:* To minimize the angular features at the forehead, use wavy bangs that blend into the temples. This softens the square forehead and draws attention to a strong jaw (Figure 4). If a beard is worn, it should be styled to slenderize the face.

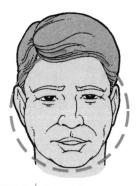

FIGURE 2 | Round face.

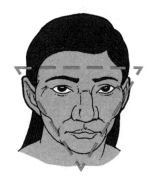

FIGURE 3 | Inverted triangular face.

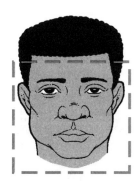

FIGURE 4 | Square face.

- *Pear-shaped:* This shape is narrow at the top and wide on the bottom (Figure 5). Create width and fullness at the top, temples, and sides to produce balance. Short, full styles are best, ending just above the jaw line where it joins the ear area. A body wave or medium-size curl perm is another way to achieve width at the top. If a beard is worn, it should be styled to slenderize the lower jaw.

- *Oblong:* The long face needs to be shortened, the angularity hidden, and the hairline never exposed (Figure 6). Blown bangs can provide a solution. A layered cut is best. A mustache helps to shorten a long face.

- *Diamond:* The aim here is to fill out the face at the temples and chin and keep hair close to the head at the widest points (Figure 7). Deep, full bangs give a broad appearance to the forehead and a fuller back section adds width. A full, square, or rounded beard would also be appropriate.

Profiles

Always be aware of the client's profile because it can influence the appropriateness of a haircut or style for that particular individual.

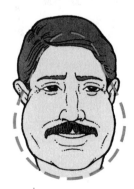

FIGURE 5 | Pear-shaped face.

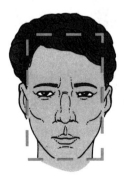

FIGURE 6 | Oblong face.

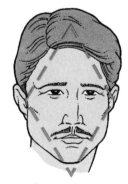

FIGURE 7 | Diamond face.

- *Straight profiles* tend to be the most balanced and can usually wear any hairstyle successfully (Figure 8).

- *Concave profiles* require a close hair arrangement over the forehead to minimize the bulge of the forehead (Figure 9).

- *Convex profiles* require some balance so arrange the top front hair over the forehead to conceal a short, receding forehead (Figure 10). A beard or goatee minimizes a receding chin.

- *Angular profiles* also have receding foreheads, but the chin tends to jut forward (Figure 11). Arrange the top front hair over the forehead to create more balance. A short beard and mustache help to minimize the protruding chin.

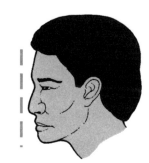

FIGURE 8 | Straight profile.

Nose Shapes

The shape of the nose influences a profile and should be studied both in profile and from a full-face view.

- *Prominent nose shapes* include a hooked nose, large nose, or pointed nose (Figure 12). Bring the hair forward at the forehead and back at the sides to minimize the prominence of the nose.

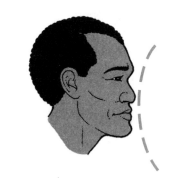

FIGURE 9 | Concave profile (prominent forehead and chin).

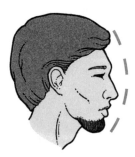

FIGURE 10 | Convex profile (receding forehead, prominent nose, and receding chin).

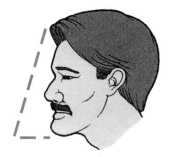

FIGURE 11 | Angular profile.

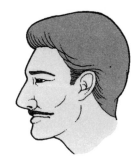

FIGURE 12 | Prominent nose.

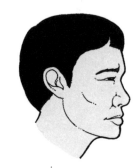

FIGURE 13 | Turned-up nose.

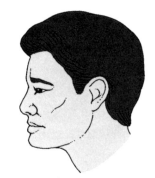

FIGURE 14 | Long neck.

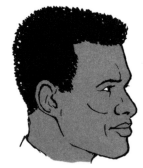

FIGURE 15 | Short neck.

▪ *Turned-up nose shapes* can usually wear shorter haircut styles because the size or heavy features associated with prominent nose shapes is not an issue (Figure 13). Experiment with combing the hair from different part lines or comb the hair back on the sides.

Neck Lengths

The length of the neck is also a factor in determining the overall shape of the haircut and style. In most cases it is advisable to follow the client's natural hairline when designing a style; however, sometimes an overly long or very short neck limits the options. The length, density, growth pattern, and natural partings of the hair should be considered when deciding on a style that best complements the client's neck length.

Long necks are minimized when the hair is left fuller or longer at the nape (Figure 14).

Short necks are best served by leaving the neck exposed to create an appearance of length (Figure 15). Work with the natural hairline and perform a tapered cut that creates an illusion of a longer nape and neck area.

FUNDAMENTALS OF HAIRCUTTING

The fundamental principles of haircutting should be thoroughly understood. The same general techniques are used in cutting, shaping, tapering, and blending men's and women's hair. The differences between the two are usually evident in the overall *design line,* the contour or shape, which includes volume, and the finished style. The fundamental principles of haircutting include the head form, basic terms used in haircutting, and different haircutting techniques.

The Head Form

In order to create consistent and successful results in haircutting, it is necessary to understand the shape of the head. Hair responds differently in different areas of the head because of the curves and changes from one section to the next. The ability to visualize these sections will assist the barber in the development of individual cutting patterns, help to eliminate technical mistakes, reduce confusion during the haircutting process, and facilitate easier checking of the final result.

When designing and cutting hair, the barber should envision the sections of the head as depicted in Figures 16 through 18. These sections include the front, top (apex), temporal, crown, sides, sideburns, back, and nape.

NOTE: The temporal section is part of the parietal ridge, which is also known as the crest, horseshoe, or hatband region of the head.

Reference points are points on the head that mark areas where the surface of the head changes or the behavior of the hair changes as a result of the surface changes. These points are used to establish proportionate design lines and contours.

■ The *parietal ridge* is also known as the crest, temporal, horseshoe, or hatband area of the head. It is the widest section of the head, starting at the temples and ending just below the crown. When a comb is placed flat against the head at the sides, the parietal ridge begins where the head starts to curve away from the

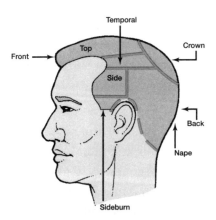

FIGURE 16 | Diagram of sections of head, side view.

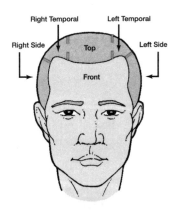

FIGURE 17 | Diagram of sections of head, front view.

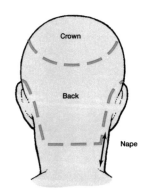

FIGURE 18 | Diagram of sections of head, back view.

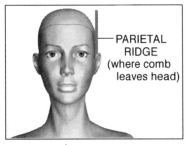

FIGURE 19 | The parietal ridge.

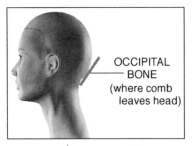

FIGURE 20 | The occipital bone.

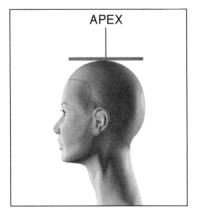

FIGURE 21 | The apex.

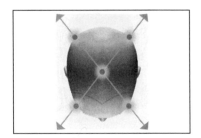

FIGURE 22 | The four corners.

comb (Figure 19). The parietal ridge is one of the most important sections of the head when cutting hair because it serves as a transition area from the top to the front, sides, and back sections.

▢ The *occipital bone* protrudes at the base of the skull. When a comb is placed flat against the nape area, the occipital begins where the head curves away from the comb (Figure 20).

▢ The *apex* is the highest point on the top of the head (Figure 21).

▢ The four corners are located by crossing two diagonal lines at the apex (Figure 22). The lines will point to the front and back corners of the head.

Basic Terms Used in Haircutting

A *line* is simply a series of connected dots that result in a continuous mark. Straight and curved lines are used in haircutting to create the shape and direction from which the hair will fall (Figure 23). The three types of straight lines used in haircutting are the horizontal, vertical, and diagonal lines (Figure 24).

▢ *Horizontal* lines are parallel to the horizon or floor and direct the eye from one side to the other. Horizontal cutting lines build weight and are used to create a one-length look and low-elevation or blunt haircut designs. These *weight lines* are usually created at the perimeter or at the occipital area of a haircut (Figures 25 and 26).

▢ *Vertical* lines are perpendicular to the floor and are described in terms of up and down. Vertical partings facilitate the projection of the hair at higher elevations while cutting. Vertical cutting lines remove weight within the cut and create layers that may be used to cut from short to long, long to short, or uniformly, depending on finger placement (Figure 27).

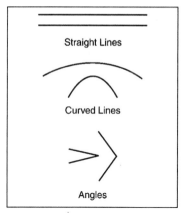

FIGURE 23 | Lines and angles.

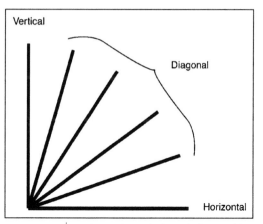

FIGURE 24 | Horizontal, vertical, and diagonal lines.

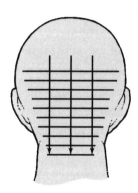

FIGURE 25 | Weight line at perimeter.

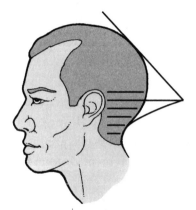

FIGURE 26 | Weight line at occipital.

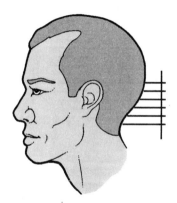

FIGURE 27 | Vertical partings facilitate layering.

■ *Diagonal* lines have a slanted direction and are used to create sloped lines at the perimeter on the design line (Figure 28). When used at the perimeter, these lines are often referred to as *diagonal forward* or *diagonal back*. Diagonal finger placement may also be used to create a stacked layered effect at the perimeter or to blend longer layers to shorter layers within a haircut.

An *angle* is the space between two lines or surfaces that intersect at a given point. Angles help to create strong, consistent foundations in haircutting and are used in two different ways. Angles can refer to the degree of elevation at which the hair is

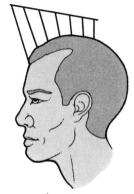

FIGURE 28 | Diagonal line within top front sections.

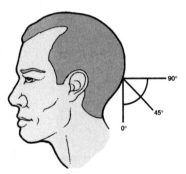

FIGURE 29 | Elevations relative to the head form.

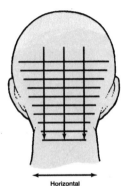

FIGURE 30 | Horizontal, zero elevation.

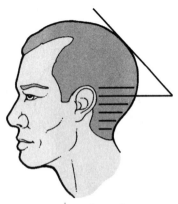

FIGURE 31 | Horizontal, 45-degree elevation.

held for cutting or to the position of the fingers when cutting a section of hair (cutting line).

Elevation is the angle or degree at which a section of hair is held from the head for cutting, *relative from where it grows*. Elevation, also known as *projection,* is the result of lifting the hair section above 0 degrees or natural fall. This projection of the hair while cutting produces graduation or layers and is usually described in terms of degrees (Figure 29).

- A low elevation of *0 degrees* produces weight, bulk, and maximum length at the perimeter of a hair design.

- To perform a 0-degree (zero elevation) cut, a *parting* is made in the section to be cut (Figure 30). After combing the hair straight down from where it grows, it is cut either against the skin (as in the nape or around-the-ear areas) or as it is held straight down between the fingers. Both stationary and horizontal traveling guides are used to create the design or perimeter line. The design line then serves as a guide for all subsequent partings that will be brought to the design (perimeter) line for cutting. This technique creates crisp, clean lines around the hairline on shorter hairstyles and achieves the standard "blunt cut" on longer hair.

- Holding the hair at *45 degrees* from where it grows is considered to be a medium elevation. Medium elevation or graduation creates layered ends or "stacking" within the parting of hair from the 0-degree distance to the 45-degree position. Movement and texture is created within the distance between the two degrees, depending on the length of the hair and the position of the angle in relation to the head form.

  Both stationary and horizontal traveling guides are used to achieve the graduated or stacked effect (Figure 31). Use of a vertical parting projected at 45 degrees, with the fingers holding the parting angled at a 45-degree diagonal, will create a *tapered* effect (Figure 32).

◘ A *90-degree* elevation is probably the most common angle used in men's haircutting. It produces layering, tapering, and blended effects. When using a 90-degree elevation, the hair is held straight out from the head from where it grows. This requires a traveling guide in order to move around the entire head. Lengths in various sections of the head can vary, but the hair will still be blended overall and considered to be a high-elevation cut.

A 90-degree *projection* can be used to create uniform layers, as depicted in Figure 33. Cutting each section of hair the same length creates *uniform* layers.

◘ To create a *tapered* effect as shown in Figure 34, the hair is held from a vertical parting and cut closer to the head form in the nape and around-the-ear areas at a 90-degree projection.

A *parting* is a smaller section of hair, usually 1/4- to 1/2-inch thick, parted off from a larger section of the hair. The use of partings is essential to maintain control of the hair in manageable

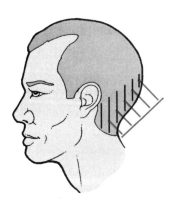

FIGURE 32 | Vertical parting with 45-degree finger placement.

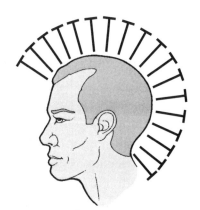

FIGURE 33 | 90-degree uniform layers.

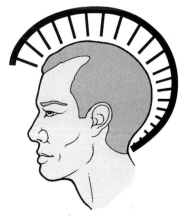

FIGURE 34 | 90-degree taper.

proportions while performing the haircut. Partings may be held horizontally, vertically, or diagonally depending on the desired effect, with a usual projection range of 0 to 180 degrees.

The *design line* is the outer perimeter line of the haircut. It may act as a guide depending on the overall design of the haircut and the method the barber uses to achieve it.

A *guide,* also known as a guideline or guide strand, is a cut that is made by which subsequent partings or sections of hair will be measured and cut. Guides are classified as being either stationary or traveling. Both types may originate at the outer perimeter (design line) of the hair, or at an interior section, usually the crown area. Most haircuts are achieved by using a combination of the two types of guides.

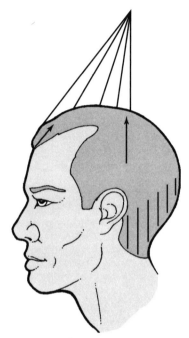

FIGURE 35 | Stationary guide.

□ A *stationary guide* is used for overall, one-length-looking designs at the perimeter, such as a solid-form blunt cut, or for maintaining the length of one section while subsequent partings are brought to it from other sections to meet it for cutting, producing either an overall long, layered effect or extra length within a section (Figure 35).

□ A *traveling guide* moves along a section of hair as each cut is made. Once the length of the initial guide has been cut, a parting is taken from in front of it or near it, combed with the original guide, and cut. Then, a new parting is taken, combed with the second parting of hair, and cut against that guide. It is this use of the previous guide to cut a subsequent parting of hair that makes it a traveling guide. Care must be taken not to recut the original or subsequent guides as the barber moves along the section. When performed properly, the traveling guide ensures even layering and blending of the hair from one section to another. Refer to Figures 33 and 34.

□ Traveling guides are used internally within the cut to create blended layers; they are also used to finish perimeter designs after the hair is cut to the desired length from one section to another. For example, although a stationary guide is used when establishing the length at the perimeter, it becomes a traveling guide when subsequent cuts are made from left to right or right to left around the head form.

Layers are produced by cutting the interior sections of the hair; they can originate from the front, top (apex), crown, or perimeter (usually the design line). Layering can be angled (shorter on top and longer at the perimeter), uniform (even throughout), or fully tapered (longer on top and shorter at the perimeter). It creates blending, fullness, and/or a feathered effect.

Tapered, or tapering, means that the hair conforms to the shape of the head and is shorter at the nape and longer in the crown and top areas. Blending of all of the hair lengths is extremely important in tapering (Figure 34).

A *weight line* refers to the heaviest perimeter area of a 0- or 45-degree cut. It is achieved by use of a stationary guide at the perimeter and may be cut in at a variety of levels on the head, depending on the style. In men's haircutting, a weight line is most often used in combination with a tapered nape area.

Texturizing is performed after the overall cut has been completed. Thinning or notching shears or razors can be used to create wispy or spiky effects within the haircut or along the perimeter.

Tension is the amount of pressure applied while combing and holding a section of hair for cutting. Tension ranges from minimum to maximum as a result of the amount of stretching employed when holding the hair between the fingers and the spacing between the teeth of the comb. For example, fine-toothed combs facilitate more tension while combing than wide-toothed combs.

□ Use maximum tension on straight hair to create precise lines.

- ☐ Use minimal to moderate tension on curly and wavy hair as the hair may dry shorter than intended if maximum tension is used.

Thinning refers to removing excess bulk from the hair.

Outlining means marking the outer perimeter of the haircut in the front (optional, depending on hair texture), in front of and over the ears, and at the sides and nape of the neck.

Over-direction creates a length increase in the design and occurs when the hair is combed away from its natural fall position, rather than straight out from the head toward a guide.

Hairstyling involves arranging the hair in a particular style, appropriately suited to the cut, and may require the use of styling aids such as hair spray, gel, tonic, oil sheen, or mousse.

During the course of your barbering career, you will be introduced to a variety of haircutting terms. Terminology for the most part depends on who is presenting the information or technique and whether or not a new word has been created in place of former terminology. The same holds true for different style names and what the latest fashion trends are. As a barber you need to be aware that cutting the hair at certain angles and elevations creates specific effects and that hairstyle trends are cyclical in nature.

Variations of design will inevitably occur, as history has a way of repeating itself in our industry. Crew cuts and boxed fades can be traced back to the years of World War II, finger waves were a hit in the 1920s, and braiding has been around since humans first walked the earth. This reinforces the fact that barbers must become proficient in the basic skills in order to adapt those skills and techniques to whatever the current trend may be.

TOOLS OF THE TRADE

Barbers should always use high-quality implements, tools, and equipment. When taken care of properly, well-tempered metal implements and electric tools will provide years of dependable service. Because a myriad of choices are available, you may want to ask an experienced barber to assist you in making appropriate selections.

Although all of the implements and tools associated with barbering will probably be used at some time or another, the principal "tools of the trade" are combs, brushes, shears, clippers, trimmers, and razors.

Combs

Combs are available in a variety of styles and sizes. The correct comb to use depends on the type of service to be performed and the individual preference of the barber. Combs are usually made of bone, plastic, or hard rubber. Because bone combs can be costly and plastic combs are not as durable as bone or rubber, most barbers prefer combs made of hard rubber. Fine-toothed combs may be used for general combing purposes, while wide-toothed combs are preferable for detangling or chemical processing. Some available comb styles are the all-purpose comb (Figure 36), the taper comb (Figure 37), the flat top comb (Figure 38), the wide-toothed comb (Figure 39), the tail comb (Figure 40) and the pick or Afro combs (Figure 41).

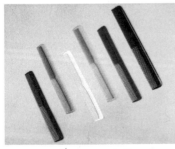

FIGURE 36 | Assorted all-purpose combs.

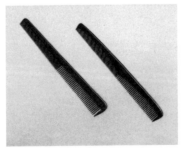

FIGURE 37 | Taper combs.

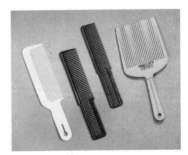

FIGURE 38 | Flat-top combs.

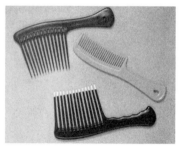

FIGURE 39 | Wide-toothed combs.

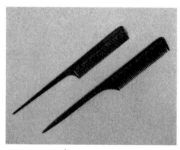

FIGURE 40 | Tail combs.

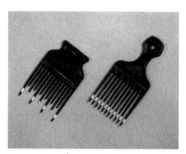

FIGURE 41 | Pick or Afro combs.

? *did you know*

Barbers can simplify their work when cutting hair by using light-colored combs on dark hair and dark-colored combs on light hair. This technique provides greater contrast between the comb and the hair, especially when employing the shear-over-comb method of cutting.

Holding the Comb

The correct manner in which to hold the comb will be dictated by the type of comb used, the service being performed, and the dexterity and comfort of the barber. Figures 42 through 45 show correct and incorrect holding positions that are often used with an all-purpose comb.

Haircutting Shears

The two types of shears generally used by barbers and barber-stylists are the French style, which has a brace for the little finger, and the German type, which does not incorporate the finger brace into the design. Barbers typically choose the French design over the German type and both are now available in ergonomically designed styles (Figure 46). Haircutting shears with detachable blades have also become very popular. The old

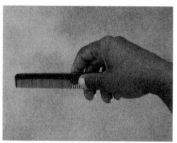

FIGURE 42 | Proper comb-holding position.

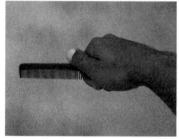

FIGURE 43 | Improper comb-holding position.

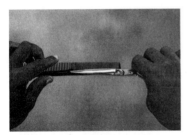

FIGURE 44 | Proper holding position for shear-over-comb cutting.

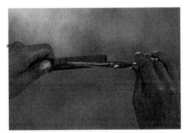

FIGURE 45 | Improper holding position for shear-over-comb cutting.

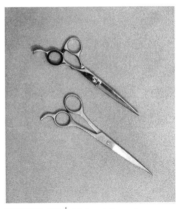

FIGURE 46 | Haircutting shears.

blades can be removed and replaced with new ones, thereby eliminating the need to send shears out to be sharpened.

Shear Facts

Shears are composed of two blades, one movable and the other stationary, fastened with a screw that acts as a pivot. Other parts of the shears are the cutting edges of the blades, two shanks, finger grip, finger brace, and thumb grip (Figure 47).

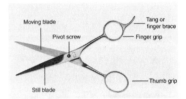

FIGURE 47 | Parts of haircutting shears.

- *Size.* Shears are available in a variety of lengths, which are measured in inches and half-inches. Most barbers prefer the 6 1/2- to 7 1/2-inch shears.

- *Grinds.* The grind of the shear refers to its cutting edge. The two main types of shear grinds are plain and corrugated. The plain grind is used most frequently and may be smooth (knife edge), medium, or coarse. The corrugated blade has imbrications. or teeth, that assist the cutting process.

- *Set.* The set of the shears refers to the alignment of the blades. This alignment is just as important as the grind of the blades because even shears with the finest cutting edges will be inferior cutting tools if the blades are not set properly.

Thinning, or serrated shears, are used to reduce hair thickness or to create special texturizing effects. They may also be called texturizing shears. One type of thinning shear has notched teeth on the cutting edge of one blade, while the other blade has a straight cutting edge. The second type has overlapping notched teeth on the cutting edges of both blades (Figure 48).

Thinning shears also differ in respect to the number of notched teeth on the cutting blade. The greater the number of notched teeth, the finer the hair strands can be cut without noticeable cut marks. The most common type used is the single serrated blade having 30 to 32 notched teeth. Recent designs include a wider notching pattern, with indentations slightly recessed in the notching teeth in order to perform alternative texturizing techniques. Thinning shears are also available with detachable blades.

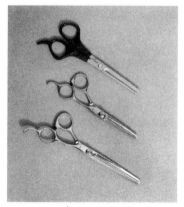

FIGURE 48 | Thinning or texturizing shears.

How to Hold Haircutting Shears

When picking up your shears in preparation for use, you will probably complete the following steps simultaneously:

1. Insert the ring finger into the finger grip of the still blade with the little finger resting on the finger brace. To ensure proper balance, brace the index finger on the shank of the still blade, approximately a half-inch from the pivot screw.

2. Next, place the tip of your thumb into the thumb grip of the moving blade. The thumb grip should be positioned halfway between the end of your thumb and the first kunckle. Avoid allowing the thumb grip to slide below the first knuckle, as you will have less control of the cutting blade. See Figures 49 and 50 for correct and incorrect finger placement and holding positions of the shears.

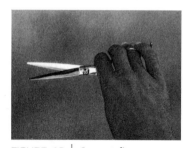

FIGURE 49 | Correct finger placement and holding position of shears.

PALMING THE SHEARS AND COMB The shears and comb should be held at all times during a haircut that requires these tools. For safety, shears need to be closed and resting in the palm while combing through the hair. This is called "palming the shears" and is achieved by slipping the thumb out of the thumb grip and simply pivoting the shear into the palm of the

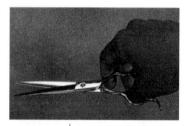

FIGURE 50 | Incorrect finger placement and holding position of shears.

hand (Figure 51). With practice, palming will become a very natural motion. Thinning or texturizing shears should be held in the same manner as regular haircutting shears.

Once the shears are palmed, the process of combing through the hair is performed with the comb in the same hand as the shears (Figure 52). After the section of hair has been combed into position for cutting, the comb is transferred to the opposite hand and palmed (Figure 53). This allows the first two fingers of that hand to be free to maintain control of the hair and the shear hand free to cut the hair section (Figure 54).

Clippers and Trimmers

Clippers and trimmers are two of the most important tools used in barbering. Clippers can be used for a variety of cutting techniques, from blending to texturizing. Trimmers, also referred to as edgers or outliners, are essential for finish and detail work.

Today's barber has a vast array of clipper styles from which to choose (Figures 55 through 57). Function, style, weight, contour, and speed are just some of the factors that should be considered when purchasing a clipper. For example, most clipper models are single speed but two-speed models are also available. Some clippers utilize a detachable blade system, whereas others

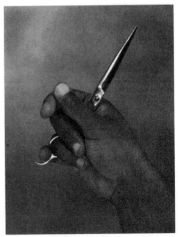

FIGURE 51 | Palming the shears.

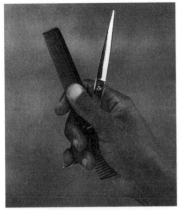

FIGURE 52 | Holding the comb and shears.

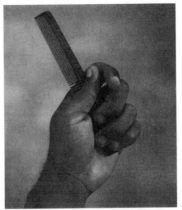

FIGURE 53 | Palming the comb.

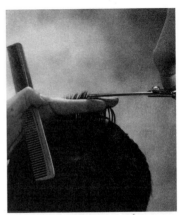

FIGURE 54 | Correct palming of comb while cutting.

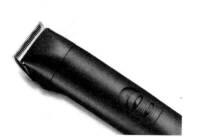

FIGURE 55 | Rotary (universal) motor clippers.

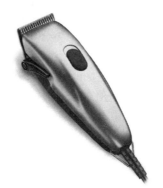

FIGURE 56 | Pivot motor clippers.

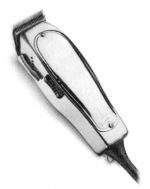

FIGURE 57 | Magnetic motor clippers.

have a single adjustable blade. Clippers with a single cutting head usually have a blade adjustment lever on the side of the unit and rely on clipper guards to vary the length of the hair being cut. Check with your local supplier for information on the different models and styles available.

Blades and Guards

Clipper *blades* are usually made of high-quality carbon steel and are available in a variety of styles and sizes (Figure 58). Some styles are intended for use with detachable-blade clipper models, and others will serve as replacement blades for certain clipper models. Blade sizes can also differ from one manufacturer to another and may not always indicate the same cutting length, so be careful when purchasing these items. A good rule of thumb is to follow the manufacturer's recommendations for the style and size of clipper blades that are appropriate for their clipper models. Manufacturers are constantly improving their clipper blades to permit faster and more precise haircutting; be on the lookout for the newest in haircutting tools.

Clipper *guards*, also known as *attachment combs*, are most often made of plastic or hard rubber and can be used with most clipper models (Figure 59). The purpose of a clipper guard is

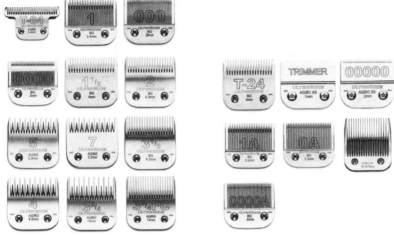

FIGURE 58 | Clipper blades.

to allow the hair to be left longer than what might be achieved from the size of the clipper blades alone. Guards do not do the actual cutting. They are simply supplemental implements that a barber may use in the pursuit of versatile techniques that can be added to his or her professional toolbox.

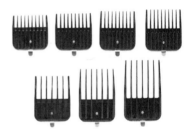

FIGURE 59 | Clipper guards.

How to Hold Clippers

The technique used by a barber to hold the clippers is most often determined by the section of the head he or she is working on. Cutting the back section will necessitate holding the clippers differently than when cutting the top section. A general rule to follow is that the clipper should always be held in a manner that permits freedom of wrist movement. Three methods of holding clippers are explained next, but you or your shop owner may use an alternative method that is equally correct.

1. When the right-handed barber holds the clippers, the thumb is placed on top of the clipper with the fingers supporting it from the underside (Figure 60). This position is usually comfortable for tapering in the nape or side areas of a haircut or when the

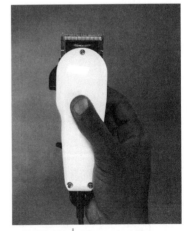

FIGURE 60 | Clipper-holding position #1.

? *did you know*

When using clippers to cut the hair, the amount of hair that remains depends on whether the hair is cut with the grain or against the grain. For example, when using a 1″ blade to cut with the grain, the approximate length of the hair that remains will be 1 1/8″ to 1 3/8″; cutting against the grain will leave the hair from 1″ to 1 1/4″ long.

i FYI

The position of the clipper blades relative to the skin and the hair's density and texture will determine the length of the hair that is left after cutting. Remember that angling the clipper blades toward the scalp or out toward the hair ends will produce different results.

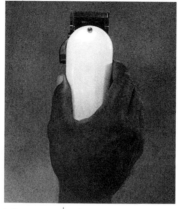

FIGURE 61 | Clipper-holding position #2.

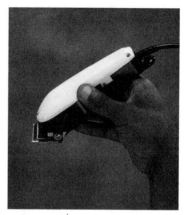

FIGURE 62 | Clipper-holding position #3.

clipper is switched to the left hand while cutting hair sections from a different direction.

2. An alternative method is to place the thumb on the left side of the unit and the fingers on the right side, with the blades pointing up (Figure 61). Like the holding position in Figure 60, some may find this a comfortable position for tapering around the hairline.

3. Figure 62 shows an alternative underhand position that may be used when working the top section of a haircut from a side-view position.

Razors

As the sharpest and closest cutting tool, razors are used for facial shaves, neck shaves, finish work around the sideburn and behind-the-ear areas, and haircutting. The razor of choice for professional barbering is the straight razor; safety razors should not be used to render professional services in the barbershop.

There are two types of straight razors: the changeable-blade straight razor and the conventional straight razor, which requires honing and stropping to maintain its cutting edge.

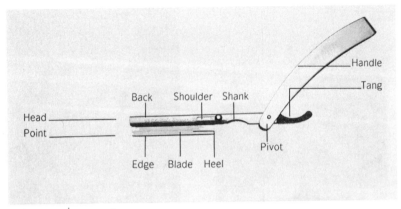

FIGURE 63 | Parts of a razor.

Both may be purchased with a razor guard. The razor guard is an attachment that is used in razor-cutting the hair. The changeable-blade razor generally looks the same as the conventional straight razor and is used in the same manner. The benefits of using the changeable-blade straight razor are the easy replacement of blades from one client service to another and the maintenance of sanitation standards in the barbershop. Also, it is usually lighter and saves time because it eliminates the need for honing and stropping. The structural parts of both conventional and changeable-blade straight razors are the head, back, shoulder, tang, shank, heel, edge, point, blade, pivot, and handle (Figure 63).

Changing the Blade

Always follow the manufacturer's directions for inserting a new blade or removing an old blade from a changeable-blade razor. Some razor models are designed with a screw mechanism that releases the blade; others require a sliding motion for blade insertion and removal. The following guidelines explain the sliding motion method of blade replacement, as illustrated in Figures 64 and 65.

1. Hold razor firmly above the joint of the handle and shank. Use the teeth of the razor guard to catch the

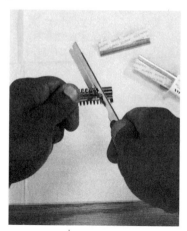

FIGURE 64 | Removing the blade.

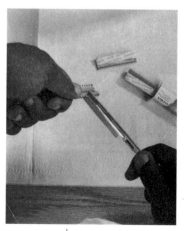

FIGURE 65 | Correct blade insertion.

blade and push it out of the razor (Figure 64). Always store used blades in a sharps container until ready for disposal.

2. To insert a new blade, position the end of the blade into the razor groove. Use the teeth of the razor guard to slide the blade in until it clicks into position (Figure 65).

NOTE: Some razor blade packaging is designed to act as a blade dispenser. The razor groove is slid over the top of the blade from the side of the dispenser until the blade is in place.

Holding the Changeable-Blade Razor

There are several methods of holding the razor, depending on the service being performed. Some of these will be covered later in this book. Others are covered in the shaving portion of *Professional Services for Men: Facial Massage and Hair Design*. However, you should practice and become familiar with the basic holding positions as follows:

1. The ball of the thumb supports the razor at the bottom of the shank between the blade and the

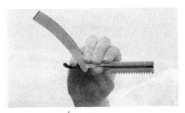

FIGURE 66 | Holding the razor properly.

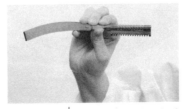

FIGURE 67 | Alternate method of holding.

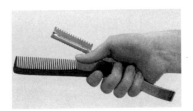

FIGURE 68 | Palming the razor and comb.

pivot. The handle is angled up, allowing the little finger to rest on the tang. Place the index finger along the back of the razor for control, with the two middle fingers resting comfortably along the top of the shank (Figure 66).

2. The razor is also held in a straightened position with the finger placement, as shown in Figure 67. This holding technique may also be used during haircutting services.

3. To palm the razor, curl in the ring finger and little finger around the handle. Hold the comb between the thumb, index, and middle fingers (Figure 68).

Lather Receptacles

Lather receptacles are containers used to hold or dispense lather for shaving. The most basic and commonly used types are the electric latherizer, the press-button-can latherizer, and the lather mug with paper lining. *Electric latherizers* are sanitary, convenient, and easy to operate (Figure 69). The sanitary and pre-heated lather coming from these modern machines impresses most clients favorably. For satisfactory performance, follow the manufacturer's instructions on their proper use and care. *Press-button-can* latherizers are convenient and sanitary, but they are not as professional as electric latherizers. *Lather mugs* are receptacles made out of glass, earthenware, rubber, or metal. When the lather mug is used, shaving soap and warm water are mixed

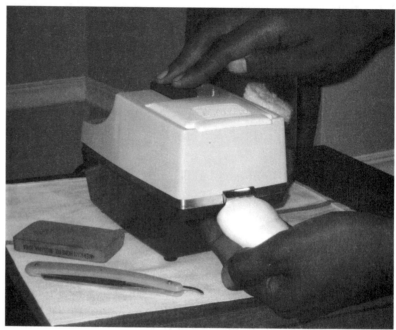

FIGURE 69 | The electric latherizer is far superior to other lather receptacles.

▽ STATE BOARD REGULATIONS

Check your state barber board rules and regulations concerning the use and disinfection of lather mugs and brushes.

thoroughly with the aid of a lather brush. Because the lather mug is exposed and collects dirt easily, it requires thorough cleansing and disinfection after each client.

Hair Removal

Hair removal methods have changed over the years. The neck duster, once a traditional implement in barbershops, is no longer a safe and sanitary option for hair removal unless sanitized after each use. Because a number of states have forbidden the use of hair dusters, other methods are now used to remove loose hair. Some methods that are in compliance with state and local health codes include:

1. A paper or cloth towel folded around the barber's hand can be used to dust off loose hair.

2. Paper neck strips can be used, but may not facilitate a very thorough dusting.

3. Small electric hand vacuums and air hoses are other options being employed.

NOTE: The electric hair vacuum provides quick cleanup service after a haircut. It can remove hair clippings and loose dandruff, and is particularly suitable for going over the forehead and around the neck and ears. Be sure to sanitize the nozzle applicator after each use and empty the container as hair accumulates within it.

HAIRCUTTING TECHNIQUES

There are several different ways to cut hair. These procedures are classified as fingers-and-shear, shear-over-comb, freehand clipper cutting, clipper-over-comb, razor-over-comb, and razor rotation. It is important to note, however, that almost every haircutting procedure requires the use of a combination of techniques and tools. The most important factors that determine the tools chosen to achieve the haircut are the client's desired outcome, the texture and density of the hair, and the barber's personal preference. As a professional barber you should be comfortable and skillful with using all the tools of the trade described thus far.

Practice the following techniques and procedures to become familiar with different methods of using your tools.

The Fingers-and-Shear Technique

The fingers-and-shear technique may be used on many hair types, from straight to curly. Three basic methods exist for using the fingers-and-shear technique: cutting on top of the fingers, cutting below the fingers, and cutting palm-to-palm.

NOTE: The blades of the shears should rest flat and flush to the fingers for these positions. Angling the shear blades may cause injury.

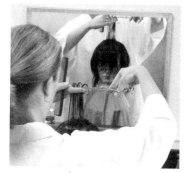

FIGURE 70 | Cutting above the fingers.

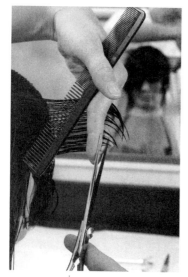

FIGURE 71 | Cutting above the fingers using a vertical parting.

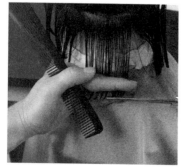

FIGURE 72 | Cutting below the fingers at the perimeter.

■ *Cutting above the fingers* is frequently used in men's haircutting to cut and blend layers in the top, crown, and horseshoe areas (Figure 70). It is also used when cutting hair that is held out at a 90-degree elevation from a vertical parting, such as the sides and back of the head form (Figure 71). Whether the barber's finger position is perpendicular to the floor or angled at 45 degrees in these sections, the cutting should be performed on the outside (on top of) the fingers.

■ *Cutting below the fingers* is most often used to create design lines at the perimeter of the haircut (Figure 72).

■ *Cutting palm-to-palm* may be preferred by some practitioners. Care must be taken not to bend the hair or to project it higher than intended from the head form when using this technique.

The Shear-over-Comb Technique

The shear-over-comb technique is used to cut the ends of the hair and is an important method used in tapering and clipper cutting. The comb is used to position the hair to be cut and is similar to holding a section of hair between the fingers. Most shear-over-comb cutting is performed in the nape, behind the ears, around the ears, and in the sideburn areas of a cut. An entire haircut, however, may also be accomplished using this method. Cutting in the nape and sideburn areas is facilitated by using vertical working panels. The cutting of areas both behind and around the ears usually requires some diagonal positioning of the comb for safety and easier access to the section. To learn the shear-over-comb technique, practice manipulating the shear and in front of a mirror (Figures 73 through 75).

1. Pick up the shears firmly with the right hand and insert the thumb into the thumb grip. Place the third

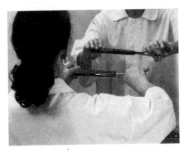

FIGURE 73 | Positioning of comb and shears.

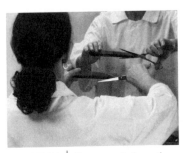

FIGURE 74 | Open and close the shears in tandem with the upward movement of the comb.

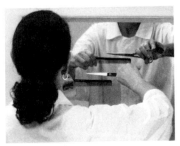

FIGURE 75 | Roll the comb using a key-turning motion.

finger into the finger grip and leave the little finger on the finger-brace of the shears. Practice opening and closing the shears, using the thumb to create the movement.

2. Pick up the comb with the left hand and place the fingers on top of the teeth with the thumb on the backbone of the comb (Figure 73).

NOTE: Start with the coarse teeth of the comb until competent at rolling the comb out and positioning the hair to be cut. After sufficient skill has been developed, use the fine teeth of the comb.

3. Practice aligning the still blade of the shears with the comb at the level where the teeth join the back, as in Figure 73. The shears and comb should be parallel to each other. Next, move the comb upward, opening and closing the shears in tandem with the movement of the comb (Figure 74). After several cutting movements, roll the teeth of the comb away from you (as if you were combing a client's hair) by using the thumb and the first two fingers in a key-turning motion (Figure 75). Master these techniques before attempting to do an actual haircut. Figures 76a and 76b illustrate the shear-over-comb technique on a mannequin.

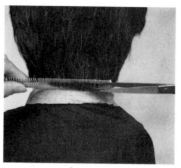

FIGURE 76A | Position the hair to be cut by rolling the comb out.

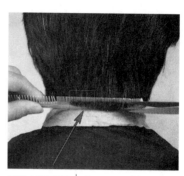

FIGURE 76B | Center point; cut to guide.

Shear-Point Tapering

Shear-point tapering is a useful technique for thinning out difficult areas of the hair caused by hollows, wrinkles, whorls, and creases in the scalp. Dark and ragged hair patches on the scalp can be minimized by this special technique. The shear-point taper is performed with the cutting points of the shears (Figures 77 and 78). Only a few strands of hair are cut at a time and then combed out. Continue cutting around the objectionable spot until it becomes less noticeable and blends in with the surrounding hair or hairline.

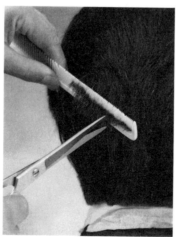

FIGURE 77 | Shear-point taper in back section.

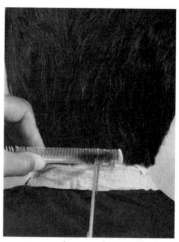

FIGURE 78 | Shear-point taper in nape area.

The Arching Technique

The arching technique is a way of marking the outer border of the haircut along the hairline at the bottom of the sideburn, in front of the ears, over the ears, and down the sides of the neck. This outlining technique is accomplished with the points of the shears or an outliner and is part of the finish work of most haircuts.

As with the other techniques in this book, the following is simply one method of performing the procedure. Figures 79 through 84 illustrate the arching technique on a mannequin.

NOTE: Before beginning the arching procedure, check to determine if one sideburn is longer than the other. Start on the side with the shortest sideburn to avoid unnecessary repetition of the procedure.

Clipper Cutting

Clippers are versatile tools that can be used in several ways to produce a variety of haircut textures and styles. The standard techniques are *freehand clipper cutting* and *clipper-over-comb* cutting. As a general rule, clipper cutting is followed up with shear

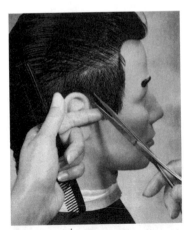

FIGURE 79 | Steady the points of the shears.

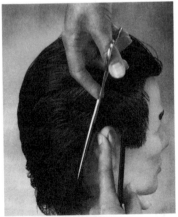

FIGURE 80 | Cut a continuous line around the ears and down the sides of the neck.

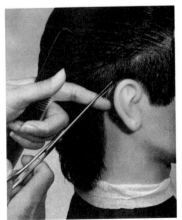

FIGURE 79 | Reverse the direction of arching.

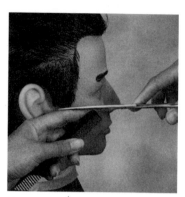

FIGURE 82 | Establish length of right sideburn.

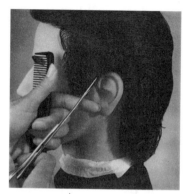

FIGURE 83 | Cut a continuous outline over the left ear and sides of the neck.

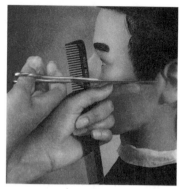

FIGURE 84 | Cut left sideburn to match the right sideburn.

and comb work to fine-tune the haircut and/or to perform the arching technique.

Directional Terms Used in Clipper Cutting

Cutting and tapering the hair with clippers can be accomplished in the following ways:

- Cutting *against the grain* is accomplished by cutting the hair in the opposite direction from which it grows (Figures 85 and 86). Taper the hair by gradually tilting the clipper until it rides on its heel.

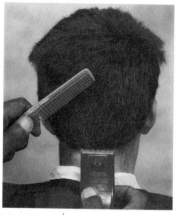

FIGURE 85 | Cutting against the grain on straight hair.

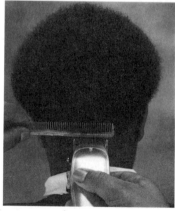

FIGURE 86 | Cutting against the grain on curly hair.

- Cutting *with the grain* means the cutting is performed in the same direction in which the hair grows (Figures 87 and 88). When using a clipper on hair that has a tight curl formation, try to cut with the grain or growth pattern. Cutting tight, curly hair against the grain clogs up the clipper blades and may leave patches or spots in the haircut.

- When cutting *across the grain* with clippers, the hair is cut neither with nor against the grain. This direction in cutting is usually performed on transition areas in the crest or side regions. (Figures 89 and 90).

- In whorl areas, or in places where the hair does not grow in a uniform manner (Figure 91), cutting the hair in a *circular motion* using clippers is advisable.

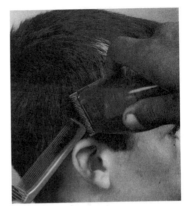

FIGURE 87 | Cutting with the grain on straight hair.

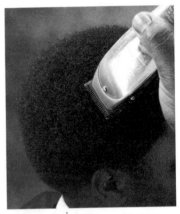

FIGURE 88 | Cutting with the grain on curly hair

Arching with a Clipper

Many barbers prefer to use an outliner or trimmer with a fine cutting edge to square off sideburns and perfect the outline around the ears and down the sides of the neck. This method of arching is efficient and precise due to the maneuverability of the smaller cutting head of the tool. If the desired result can be accomplished with the standard clipper, that method is equally acceptable (Figures 92 and 93).

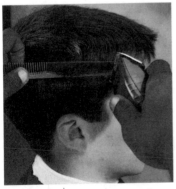

FIGURE 89 | Cutting across the grain on straight hair.

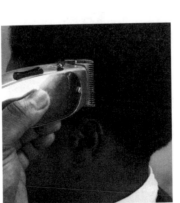

FIGURE 90 | Cutting across the grain on curly hair.

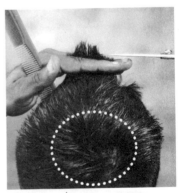

FIGURE 91 | Whorl in crown area in straight hair.

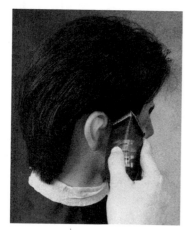

FIGURE 92 | Arching with clipper in front of the ear.

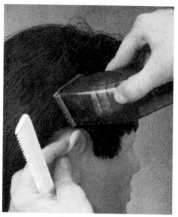

FIGURE 93 | Arching with clipper around ear.

Freehand and Clipper-over-Comb Cutting

Freehand clipper cutting requires a steady hand and consistent use of the comb or hair pick while cutting. The use of the comb or pick is important for two reasons: First, both implements put the hair into a position to be cut, and second, both implements help to remove the excess hair cut from the previous section. This provides the barber with a clear view of the results of the previous work and any areas that may need reblending.

A true freehand clipper cutting technique tends to be used on two extremes of hair length: (1) very short straight, wavy, and curly lengths in which little clipper-over-comb work is performed; and (2) longer, very curly hair lengths that require more sculpting (Figures 94 and 95).

For short hair styles, clippers with detachable blades range from size 0000 (close to shaving) to size 3 1/2, which leaves the hair almost 1/2-inch long. Detachable blades should not be confused with clipper attachment combs, most commonly known as *guards*. Guards are placed on top of a clipper blade, allowing for more hair length to remain while cutting.

NOTE: The use of guards is not considered to be a form of freehand clipper cutting, nor are guards generally acceptable for state board practical examinations.

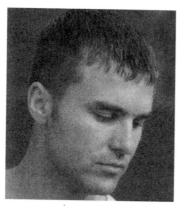

FIGURE 94 | Finished freehand clipper cut on straight hair.

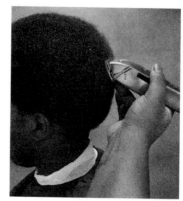

FIGURE 95 | Freehand clipper cutting.

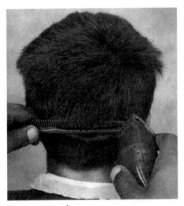

FIGURE 96 | Clipper over comb on straight hair.

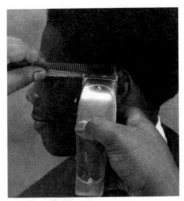

FIGURE 97 | Clipper over comb on curly hair.

Freehand clipper cutting is also used for tightly curled hair when a natural look is the desired result. Because most tightly curled hair grows up and out of the scalp, rather than falling to one side or another as with straighter hair types, the hair texture lends itself to being picked out and put into position for freehand clipper cutting. Cutting this type of hairstyle requires a keen eye for haircut balance, shape, and proportion as the hair is sculpted into the desired form.

Clipper-over-comb cutting can be used to cut the entire head or to blend the hair from shorter tapered areas to longer-haired areas such as the top, crest, or occipital. Much like the shear-over-comb technique, the comb places the hair in a position to be cut and utilizes the same blending principles (Figures 96 and 97). Freehand clipper cutting, clipper-over-comb, and fingers-and-shear work are techniques frequently used to perform a single haircut.

▷ procedure no. 1

Clipper Cutting

This procedure will involve clipper-over-comb cutting and standard freehand clipper cutting using an all-purpose comb.

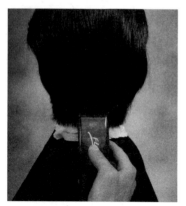

FIGURE 98 | Hold clipper to permit freedom of wrist movement.

1   How to hold the clipper and comb for *clipper-over-comb cutting:*

a. Pick up the clipper with the dominant hand.

b. Place the thumb on the top left side and fingers underneath along the right side of the clipper. Hold it firmly, but lightly, to permit freedom of wrist movement (Figure 98).

c. Use the largest numbered detachable clipper blade or fully open the adjustable blade clipper.

d. Begin in the center of the nape area and comb the hair down with the opposite hand (Figure 99).

e. With the teeth of the comb pointing upward, comb into a section of hair at the hairline, rolling the comb out toward you as in Figure 100.

f. Use the clipper to cut the hair section to the desired length. Comb through, check, and begin the next section to the right or left of center.

2   Clipper-over-comb: cutting the nape area:

a. For a gradual, even taper from shorter to longer in each section of hair, roll the comb out to put the hair in a position to be cut.

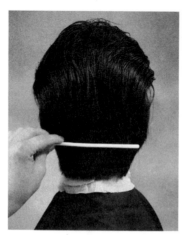

FIGURE 99 | Begin in the center of the nape and comb the hair down.

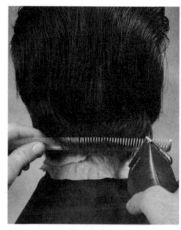

FIGURE 100 | Roll the comb out to put the hair in a position to be cut.

b. Gradually taper the hair from the hairline to an inch or two above the hairline. Do not taper higher than the occipital for this procedure, or cut into the hair along the sides of the neck at this point (Figure 101).

3 Clipper-over-comb—cutting the sides:

a. Begin in the front of the ear and position the comb parallel to the hairline. Roll the hair out at about a 45-degree projection and cut (Figure 103). Follow the forward curve of the hairline around the ear.

b. Bend the ear forward and use the same projection technique to continue cutting along the hairline to meet the hairline at the topmost part at the back of the ear.

4 Clipper-over-comb—cutting behind the ears:

a. The guide around the ears and at the corner of the neck should be visible.

b. Place the comb parallel to the hairline on a diagonal, roll the comb out, and blend from the guide at the back of the ear to the nape corner (Figures 104a and 104b). The hair in the tapered areas should blend from the nape to the side of the neck, and around the ear.

5 How to hold the clipper for freehand clipper cutting:

a. Pick up the clipper with the dominant hand.

b. Place the thumb on the top left side and fingers underneath along the right side of the clipper. Hold it firmly, but lightly, to permit freedom of wrist movement. Depending on the section of the head form being cut, the holding position will change for comfort and access to the area.

c. Use the largest-numbered detachable clipper blade or fully open the adjustable-blade clipper.

d. Begin in the center of the nape area and comb the hair down with the opposite hand.

FYI

When tapering with the clipper-over-comb technique, be sure to tilt the comb away from the head to create a blended taper from shorter to longer sections (Figure 102).

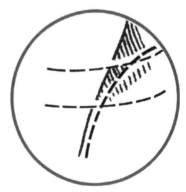

FIGURE 101 | Continue clipper-over-comb cutting to the occipital area.

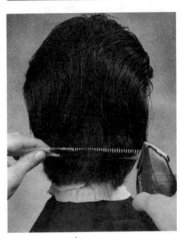

FIGURE 102 | When tapering with a clipper, be sure to tilt the comb away from the head to create a blended taper from shorter to longer sections.

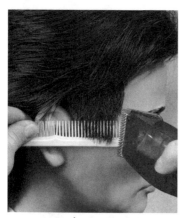

FIGURE 103 | Position the comb at the hairline and roll out to 45 degrees.

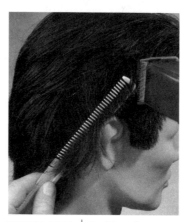

FIGURE 104A | Position the comb parallel to the hairline.

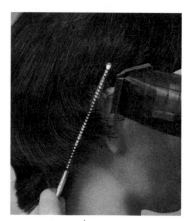

FIGURE 104B | Continue cutting to the corner of the nape.

e. Palm the comb and steady the clipper with the tip of the index finger of the opposite hand.

6 Freehand clipper cutting—the nape area:

a. Begin with the clipper blades open. With the teeth of the bottom blade placed flat against the skin at the center of the nape hairline, lightly guide the clipper upward into the hair 1/4 to 1/2 inch above the hairline (Figure 105).

b. For a gradual, even taper from shorter to longer hair, gradually tilt the blade away from the head so that the clipper rides on the heel of the bottom blade (Figure 106). Do not taper higher than the occipital for this procedure. Gradually taper the hair only an inch or two above the hairline.

NOTE: The style will determine the point on the head at which the tapered area is blended into longer hair. Very short styles, such as butch and crew cuts, have a high taper and are blended in the crest areas; longer

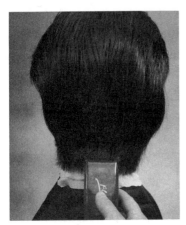

FIGURE 105 | Guide the clipper blades through the ends of the hair.

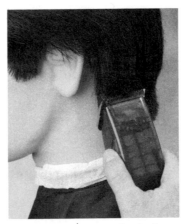

FIGURE 106 | Gradually tilt the clipper blades away from the head.

styles may be blended at or just below the occipital. There are as many variations as there are heads of hair to cut.

   c. Do not move the clipper into the hair too fast as it may have a tendency to jam the clipper blades and pull the hair.

   d. After tapering one short strip of hair, comb it down, check the results, and start tapering the section to the right or left of center.

7 Freehand clipper cutting—the sides:

   a. Begin at the front of the ear at the hairline and comb the hair down. Tilt the clipper at about a 45-degree angle so that the first few teeth of the blades will be used for cutting the curve around the ear.

   b. Bend the ear forward and continue cutting along the hairline, meeting the top of the hairline at the side of the neck.

8 Freehand clipper cutting—behind the ears:

   a. The guide around the ears and at the corner of the neck should be visible.

b. Comb the hair down and blend from the nape corner to the guide at the back of the ear. The hair in the tapered areas should blend from the nape to the side of the neck and around the ear.

▷ procedure no. 2

Clipper Cutting Tightly Curled Hair

1   Hold the clipper as for freehand clipper cutting.

2   Use a pick or Afro comb to comb the hair up and outward from the scalp.

3   If the hair is too thick or too tightly curled to use an all-purpose comb while cutting, use a wide-tooth comb to practice the clipper-over-comb technique, as performed on the model in Figure 97.

4   When the clipper-over-comb technique has been completed, practice the freehand clipper cutting method shown in Figure 95.

Be guided by your instructor as to where to begin the clipper cut and the order of the subsequent sections. Some barbers prefer to start in the center of the nape area, whereas others work from right to left or left to right. As long as the hair is tapered evenly, all methods are equally correct.

Clipper Cut Styles

Variations of the basic clipper cut styles have been around since the hand clipper was invented. Flat tops, crew cuts, and the Quo Vadis are three of the most popular styles that have stood the test of time and cyclical haircut trends.

Flat tops are very short on the sides and in the back areas, as are crew cuts. Flat tops are traditionally slightly longer in the front and crest sections and flat across the top of the head form. The top of the crest area should look squared off when viewed from the front. Variations of the style and length of the top section will be determined by the client's preference, hair texture, and hair density. Clippers or shears or use of both tools may be used to cut a flat top (Figure 107).

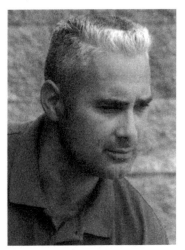

FIGURE 107 | Flat-top style.

▷ procedure no. 3

Cutting the Flat Top

Suggested procedures for cutting the flat top are as follows:

1   Stand behind the client. The hair at the crown is cut flat to about 1/4 to 1/2 inch in length, 1 inch in depth, and 2 to 3 inches in width.

2   Stand in front of the client. Position the comb flat across the front center area, cutting the hair to a length of 1 to 1 1/2 inches, depending on the client's preference. This cutting area will span the width of the client's top section. Cut straight across from side to side.

3   Ask the client if the front hair is the desired length. If it is not, then cut the hair to the desired height.

4   Complete all finish work such as arching and the neck shave.

Crew cuts are also referred to as the *short pomp* or *brush cut*. The length of hair on the sides and back of the head usually determines the crew cut style, as described in the following list:

- ◻ Short sides and back: short crew cut.
- ◻ Semishort sides and back: medium crew cut.
- ◻ Medium sides and back: long crew cut.

Generally, the back and sides are cut first and relatively high to the bottom of the crest area. The hair on top is then combed from front to back to make it stand up, followed by blending the tapered area to the crest and top sections. Because the top section should be smooth and almost flat, use a wide-toothed comb to provide a level guide. Begin cutting in the front to the desired length and cut back toward the crown. This section should be graduated in length from the front hairline to the back part of the crown. Repeat the procedure until the top section has been cut. When viewed from the front, the top section should blend with the top of the crest, with a slight curvature to conform to the contours of the head. Use the shears and comb to smooth out any uneven spots left by the clipper work.

The brush cut is a variation of the crew cut and is popular with young men because it requires the least attention. The sides and back areas are cut as for a short crew cut, but the hair on top is cut the same length all over, about 1/4 to 1/2 inch, and follows the contours of the head.

The Quo Vadis is a popular haircut style that is suitable for very curly hair. The main objective with this haircut is to achieve an even and smooth cut over the entire head. Because the hair is cut close to the scalp, clipper lines and patches are readily noticeable. Be guided by the natural hair growth pattern and cut with the grain to avoid gaps. Outline and taper the nape area with a #000 clipper blade and then use a #1 clipper blade over the rest of the head.

Basic Tapering and Blending Areas

To simplify the clipper or shear cutting procedures, the primary tapering and blending areas of haircut styles may be identified as belonging to one of four basic classifications: long cuts and trims, medium lengths, semishort lengths, and short cuts. A variety of hairstyles, such as the fade and bilevel, can be created from these basic classifications to suit the client's tastes and desires.

Long haircut styles and trims usually require the least amount of clipper tapering. Tapering is performed from the nape hairline to just above the bottom of the ear and below the occipital using the fingers-and-shear, shear-over-comb, or clipper-over-comb techniques (Figure 108). An outliner or trimmer is used to remove fine hair at the nape and along the sides of the neck.

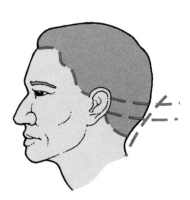

FIGURE 108 | Taper area for longer hair style.

Sideburns and over-the-ear areas are shortened using the shear-over-comb method along the natural hairline and then outlined with trimmers and/or razor.

Medium-length styles do not usually have a scalped appearance, although the hair is cut closer to the head than in longer styles (Figure 109). Clipper cutting at the nape should be performed with the clipper tilted on its heel until reaching a point about midway to the ears. In the sideburn areas, the taper should end no higher than the tops of the ears. An outliner or razor is used at the nape hairline.

Semishort styles usually require tilting the clipper back off the hair when the top of the ear areas are viewed from the back section. The hair in the back may be left slightly longer than on the sides. In the sideburn areas, the clipper tapers out at about the top of the ears. When cutting around the ears, remove about 1/2 inch from the hairline, then use an outliner to trim the sideburns and around the ear areas (Figure 110).

Short haircut styles usually require cutting up to the crest area and then gradually tilting the heel of the clipper back as the clipper is brought up until it runs off the curve of the head. This movement is repeated all the way around the head form. An outliner is used to taper the sideburns and nape (Figure 111).

The *fade style* derives its name from the fact that the hair at the nape and sides is cut extremely close, becoming gradually

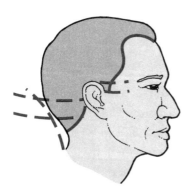

FIGURE 109 | Taper area for medium-length style.

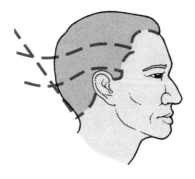

FIGURE 110 | Taper area for semishort style.

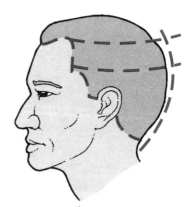

FIGURE 111 | Taper area for short styles.

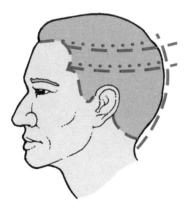

FIGURE 112 | Taper area for a fade style.

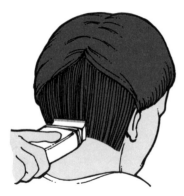

FIGURE 113 | Taper area for a bilevel style.

longer in the crest and lower crown areas and longest at the top. Hence, it fades to nothing at the hairline.

This cut requires close cutting from the nape to the bottom of the crest or horseshoe area. The sides are cut to the temporal region using the next-longer clipper blade, or one that will taper in the crest area to the top section. The top section is cut and blended to the crest (Figure 112). To gradually blend the fine clipper taper with the longer clipper taper, tilt the heel of the clippers, moving with and across the grain as necessary.

A *bilevel style* cut is most often achieved with clippers and shears. The clipper is used to cut the nape and sides to the desired length (Figure 113). The top is either layered and texturized or cut to one length using a weight line. The weight line may vary in style lengths.

For a medium-length style, the top, crown, and crest area hair is sectioned off and secured with a hair clip. Clipper cutting is performed up to the occipital area in the back and on the sides to the bottom of the crest. A horizontal parting is taken from the secured hair to establish a design/guide line. The hair is cut at 0 degrees until all the partings are cut. Using the design line as a guide, the hair is projected at 45 or 90 degrees to produce layers, if desired. Clipper cutting for a shorter length, bilevel style usually requires cutting higher into the temporal region with slight blending to the top section.

Popular Sideburn Lengths

When trimming or redesigning the length of sideburns, every effort should be made to make sure that the sideburns appear even in length. When seen in profile, the client's ear, eye, or other anatomical feature may be used as a general guide for trimming the sideburns. However, *always check the length of both sideburns by facing the client toward the mirror.* No one's face is truly symmetrical and differences will be noticed when viewing the client from the front. In addition, check to see that the thickness (density) of the sideburns complements the facial shape and hairstyle (Figures 114 through 118).

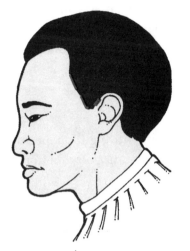

FIGURE 114 | Short sideburn.

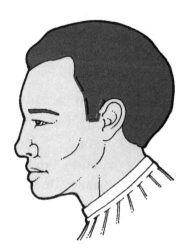

FIGURE 115 | Medium sideburn.

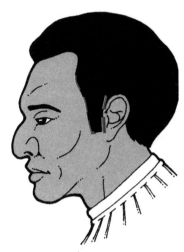

FIGURE 116 | Long sideburn.

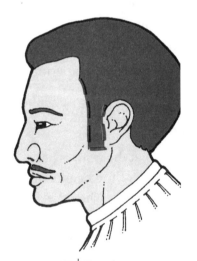

FIGURE 117 | Extra-long sideburn.

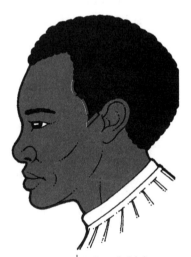

FIGURE 118 | Pointed sideburn.

Razor Cutting

Razor cutting provides an opportunity for the barber to create a variety of different effects in the hair (Figure 119). It is especially suitable for thinning, shortening, tapering, blending, or feathering specific areas and can help make resistant hair textures more manageable. For client comfort and a precise cut, the hair should

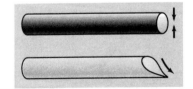

FIGURE 119 | Shear cut and razor cut strands.

always be clean and damp. As always, the barber must consider the client's styling wishes, features, head shape, facial contour, and hair texture. The technique of handling a razor should be mastered completely before attempting to use it to cut a client's hair.

Razor Stroking and Combing

Proper stroking of the razor and combing during the tapering process are of utmost importance in razor cutting. It is better to taper a little at a time than to taper too much.

- *Arm and hand movements:* Some barbers prefer the arm movement, in which the razor stroking and combing is done with stiff arms, using the elbows as a hinge. Others use both wrist and arm movements. This is a matter of preference. The barber should develop a technique best suited to the individual and that gives the desired results.

- *Razor taper-blending:* Razor cutting is thought by some barbers to be the best technique to use for tapering and blending the hair. The cutting action of the razor permits a smoother blend than that usually accomplished with shears and/or clippers.

  Light taper-blending requires that the razor is held almost flat against the surface of the hair. Note the small amount of hair that is cut when the blade is only slightly tilted and very little pressure is used (Figure 120).

  Heavier taper-blending is performed with the razor held up to 45 degrees from the surface of the hair strand. As the razor is tilted higher and a little more pressure is used, the depth of the cut increases (Figure 121).

  Terminal blending means that the angle of the razor blade is increased to almost 90 degrees. Short sawing strokes are used. Other terms used for terminal blending are *hair-end tapering* and *blunt cutting* (Figure 122).

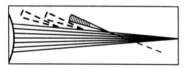

FIGURE 120 | Light taper-blending.

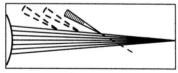

FIGURE 121 | Heavier taper-blending.

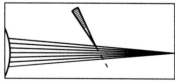

FIGURE 122 | Terminal blending.

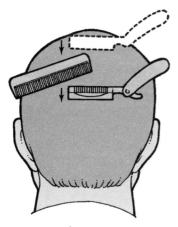

FIGURE 123 │ Crown area: razor and comb coordination.

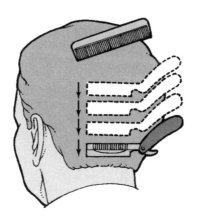

FIGURE 124 │ Nape area: razor and comb coordination.

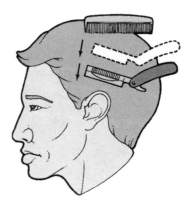

FIGURE 125 │ Side areas: razor and comb coordination.

- *Razor and comb coordination:* Razor stroking and combing are done in a continuous movement. The razor tapers while the comb removes the cut hair and recombs the section for the next stroke or strokes (Figures 123 through 125).

Hair Textures and Razor Cutting

- *Coarse, thick hair* requires more strokes and heavier tapering than other textures. The first strip of hair is combed, followed by three razor strokes and followed again with the comb. The comb removes the cut hair and recombs the hair, allowing the barber to see how much hair has been cut. It also helps to keep the guide in view for use in tapering the next strip (Figures 126 through 128).

- *Medium-textured hair* requires fewer razor strokes and lighter pressure than coarse, thick hair, as pictured in Figures 129 through 132.

- *Fine hair* typically does not have any bulk to remove; however, the razor may be used to blend hair ends to achieve a particular hairstyle. Stroking of the razor is usually lighter than that used for medium-textured hair.

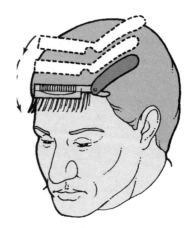

FIGURE 126 │ Top area: Consideration must be given to the hairstyle to be created. The stroking and the pressure of the razor largely depend upon the amount of hair to be removed to achieve the finished hairstyle.

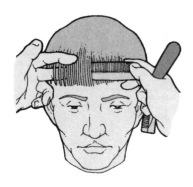

FIGURE 127 | Front hair: To equalize the length of long and uneven front hair, pick up the hair with the comb in the right hand. Hold the hair straight out between the middle and index fingers of the left hand.

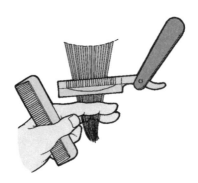

FIGURE 128 | Palm the comb to the left hand. Hold the razor at an angle, and with short, sawing strokes cut the hair to the desired length.

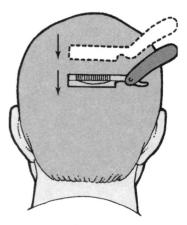

FIGURE 129 | Crown area: two long strokes are used.

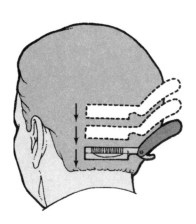

FIGURE 130 | Nape area: Three short strokes are used.

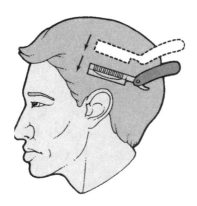

FIGURE 131 | Left and right sides of the head: Two short strokes may be used.

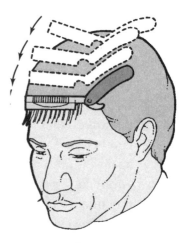

FIGURE 132 | Top area: The stroking and pressure of the razor in this area are the same as for the sides and back area.

Terms Associated with Razor Cutting

Removing weight can be accomplished by holding a parting of damp hair out from the head with the fingers positioned at the end of the section. Place the razor flat to the hair and gently stroke the razor to remove a thin sheet of hair from the section. This technique tapers the ends of the hair (Figure 133).

Freehand slicing can be used in the midshaft of a section or at the ends of the hair. The hair is combed out from the head and held between the fingers, where the tip of the razor will be used to slice out pieces of hair. This technique releases weight from the subsection and allows for more movement within the hairstyle. When used to cut the design line, freehand slicing the ends helps to create soft perimeters (Figures 134 and 135).

Razor-over-comb cutting is slightly different from shear or clipper-over-comb techniques in which the comb is used to project the hair into a position for cutting. In razor-over-comb cutting, the razor is held in the freehand position and situated just above the comb as it follows the comb's downward direction through the hair (Figure 136). Short, precise strokes with medium pressure are applied to the surface of the hair. This technique is often used to taper nape areas or to soften weight lines.

Razor rotation is performed by using a rotating motion with the comb and razor as the hair is being cut. In the first movement, the razor follows the comb through the hair. Then the comb follows the razor, and so on (Figure 137).

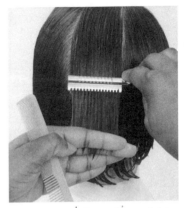

FIGURE 133 | Removing weight with freehand slicing.

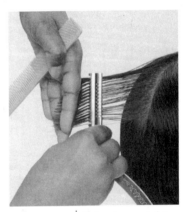

FIGURE 134 | Releasing weight from a subsection.

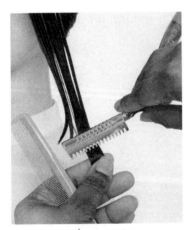

FIGURE 135 | Establishing a design line at the perimeter.

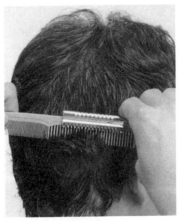

FIGURE 136 | Razor-over-comb technique.

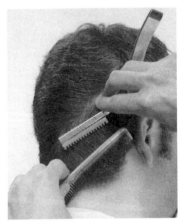

FIGURE 137 | Razor rotation.

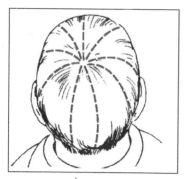

FIGURE 138 | Umbrella effect.

Hair Sectioning for Razor Haircutting

There are several effective ways to section the hair for razor cutting. These include the two-section, three-section, four-section, and five-section methods. All methods begin by combing the hair into the umbrella effect, which is created by combing the hair into natural directions from the crown (Figure 138). Be guided by your instructor.

- *Two sections.* First, part the hair from ear to ear across the crown. All hair in front of the part is combed forward. All hair behind or below the part is combed down (Figure 139).

- *Three sections.* First, part the hair from ear to ear across the crown. All top and side hair is combed forward. Then make a vertical part from the crown to the nape. Each of these subsections is combed toward the sides. In the nape area where there is no part, comb the hair down (Figure 140).

- *Four sections.* Add one more section to the previous three sections. Make a top center part and comb each side down (Figure 141).

- *Four sections, alternate method.* First, part the hair from ear to ear across the crown. Second, section the right side from the center of the right eyebrow to the crown and comb down. Make another section on the left side

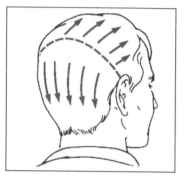

FIGURE 139 | Two sections.

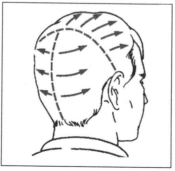

FIGURE 140 | Three sections.

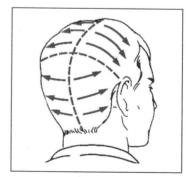

FIGURE 141 | Four sections.

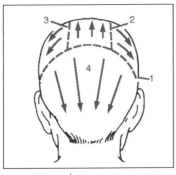

FIGURE 142 | Four sections (alternate method).

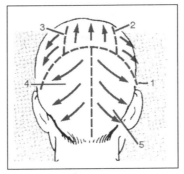

FIGURE 143 | Five sections.

from the center of the left eyebrow to the crown and comb down. Comb all back hair down (Figure 142).

- *Five sections.* Sectioning is the same as the alternate four section, except that the back section is divided in two and combed as indicated by the arrows in Figure 143.

▷ procedure no. 4

Razor Cutting

A *pattern for cutting* needs to be established by the barber so that there is a plan to follow. In this book, one basic plan is followed. Other procedures may be different, but equally correct.

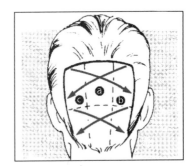

FIGURE 144 | Back.

1   Back part of head (Figure 144):
   a. Downward
   b. Top right to left, downward
   c. Top left to right, downward

2   Right side of head (Figure 145):
   a. Downward
   b. Toward the back
   c. Toward the face

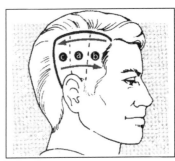

FIGURE 145 | Sides.

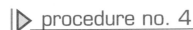

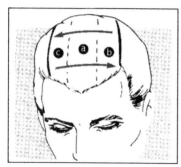

FIGURE 146 | Top.

3 Left side of head:
   a. Downward
   b. Toward the back
   c. Toward the face

4 Top hair (Figure 146):
   a. Crown to forehead
   b. Top left side
   c. Top right side

For the best results in razor cutting the hair must be clean and damp. Avoid tapering too close to the hair part or the scalp. Tapering the hair too closely to the hair part will cause the hair to stand up, making the part look ragged. Coarse hair that is cut too closely to the scalp will have short, stubby hair ends that will protrude through the top layer. Avoid overtapering the hair; it is difficult to correct a haircut after too much hair has been removed.

Razor-Cutting Safety Precautions

◻ Handle the razor properly, keeping it closed whenever not in use.

◻ Be aware of the people around you when working with any sharp tool or implement. A careless motion can cause injury to yourself or others. Do not annoy or distract anyone who is in the process of performing a service.

◻ Purchase and use only good-quality haircutting implements.

◻ Use changeable-blade razors and dispose of used blades in a sharps container.

◻ Replace dull razor blades, during a cut if necessary, as a dull blade will pull the hair and cause pain or discomfort to the client. Dull blades will also influence the quality of the haircut.

Hair Thinning and Texturizing

Hair thinning is used to reduce the bulk or weight of the hair. The barber can use thinning (serrated) shears, regular shears, clippers, or a razor for this purpose. Regardless of the tool used to perform the procedure, some general rules to follow when removing bulk from the hair are as follows:

- Make a careful observation of the hair to determine the sections that require some reduction in bulk or weight and cut accordingly.

- Avoid cutting top surfaces of the hair where visible cutting lines can be seen.

- Part off and elevate the hair to be cut to avoid cutting too deeply into the section.

- Avoid cutting too closely to the scalp or part lines.

Removing Bulk

When thinning with serrated shears the hair parting is combed and held between the index and middle finger. The shears are placed about midshaft on the strands and a cut is made (Figure 147). If another cut is necessary it should be made about 1 inch from the first cut. Do not cut twice in the same place.

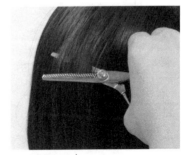

FIGURE 147 | Removing bulk midshaft with thinning shears.

Two slicing methods can be used to remove bulk with regular shears. Figure 148 shows the slicing technique performed on the surface of the hair. A second method is to part off a vertical section of hair and elevate between 45 and 90 degrees. Standing from the side of the hair projection, open the shears and position the parting close to the pivot. Carve through the partings with a curving motion that removes hair from the underportion of the parting as the motion is continued to the hair ends (Figure 149).

Another method that can be used to remove bulk with regular shears involves *slithering*. In this procedure a thin parting of hair is held between the fingers. The shears are positioned for cutting and an up-and-down sliding motion along the parting is

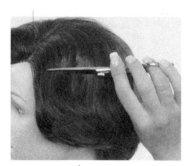

FIGURE 148 | Slicing on hair surface to remove bulk.

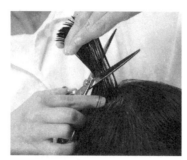

FIGURE 149 | Carving with shears to remove bulk.

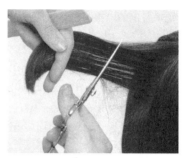

FIGURE 150 | Slithering midshaft to remove bulk.

combined with a slight closing of the shears each time they are moved toward the scalp (Figure 150).

Removing Weight from the Ends

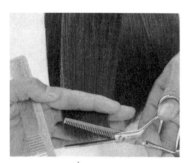

FIGURE 151 | Removing weight from the ends.

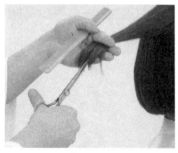

FIGURE 152 | Notching.

Removing weight from the ends helps to taper the perimeter of graduated and blunt haircuts. This can be accomplished using thinning shears by elevating the section and placing the shears at an angle as the cuts are made or by using the comb to put the hair into position for cutting (Figure 151).

To remove weight with regular shears, *point cutting* or *notching* can be used to reduce weight in the ends of the hair. For either technique, a parting is held between the fingers and the tips of the shears are used on a vertical angle to create points or notches in the hair (Figure 152).

Both clippers and razors can be used to remove weight from the ends of the hair. Use a clipper-over-comb technique to put the hair ends in a position to be cut and position the clipper blades under the ends of the hair. Use a *reverse* rotation technique with the clipper to comb through and cut the ends from one section to another. The razor-over-comb technique should be used when lightening hair ends with a razor.

Haircut Finish Work: Shaving the Outline Areas

The performance of a neck shave and the shaving of the outline areas as a feature of the haircut service contribute to the appearance of the finished cut and provide the client with a true barbershop experience. At one time, it was the barber's standard operating procedure to finish a haircut with these shaving services. Yet, while many traditionally oriented barbers still perform neck and outline shaves, others in the industry have exchanged razors for outliners or trimmers on a more or less permanent basis. This is a trend that should be changed by today's barber, as the traditional barbering services are once more being sought by consumers.

The traditional *neck shave* consists of shaving the sides of the neck and across the nape with a razor (see Figures 153 through 155). The *outline* consists of the sideburn areas and around the ears and nape area; with African-American styles, the front hairline is often included.

The following *preparation steps* should be used in the performance of these shaving services:

1. Remove all cut hair from around the head and neck with a clean towel, tissues, or hair vacuum.

2. Loosen the chair cloth and remove the neck strip used during the haircut. Be careful that loose clippings do not fall down the client's neck or shirt.

3. Pick up the chair cloth at the lower edge, fold it upward to the top edge, and gather the four corners together. Remove the chair cloth carefully so that cut hair does not fall on the client. Turn away from the chair and drop the lower edge of the chair cloth, giving a slight shake to dislodge all cut hair.

4. Replace the chair cloth, resting it a few inches away from the neck so that it does not touch the client's skin.

5. Spread a terry cloth or paper towel straight across the shoulders and tuck it loosely around the client's neck. Secure the chair cloth and fold the towel over the neckband. The drape should be loose enough to

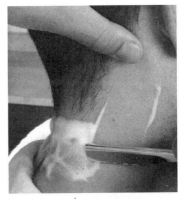

FIGURE 153 | Neck shave on the right side with freehand stroke.

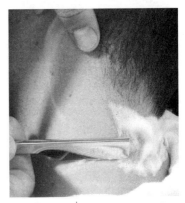

FIGURE 154 | Neck shave on the left side with reverse backhand stroke.

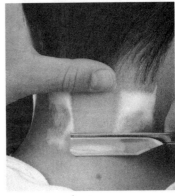

FIGURE 155 | Neck shave in the nape area with freehand stroke.

permit easy access to the neck area. Tuck a towel or neck strip into the neckband of the drape for wiping the razor.

▷ procedure no. 5

Shaving the Outline Areas

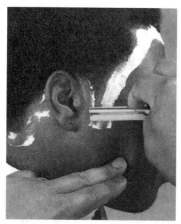

FIGURE 156 | Step 1. Apply lather around hairline.

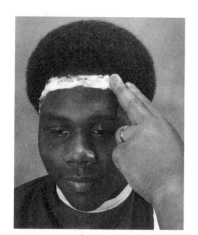

FIGURE 157 | Step 2: Shave sideburn to desired length.

1　Apply a light coating of lather at the hairline of the sideburns, around and over the ears, the front hairline, down the sides of the neck, and across the nape. *Apply lather to the back of the neck and/or the front hairline of the client only if these areas are to be shaved.* Rub the lather in lightly with the balls of the fingers or thumb. (Figure 156).

2　Shaving the right side:
  a. Hold the razor for a freehand stroke.
  b. Place the left thumb on the scalp above the point of the razor and gently stretch the skin under the razor.
  c. Shave the sideburn to the desired length (Figure 157).
  d. Shave around the ear at the hairline and straight down the side of the neck, using the freehand stroke with the point of the razor. Be careful not to shave into the hairline at the nape of the neck (Figures 158 through 160).

3　Shaving the left side
  a. Hold the razor as in the reverse backhand stroke.
  b. Place the left thumb on the scalp above the razor point, and gently stretch the skin under the razor.
  c. Shave the sideburn to the proper length using the reverse-backhand or backhand stroke (Figure 161).
  d. Shave around the ear at the hairline, using the freehand stroke (Figure 162a).

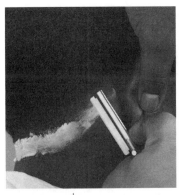

FIGURE 158 | Stretch skin and shave in front of ear.

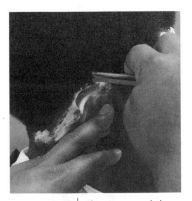

FIGURE 159 | Shave around the ear.

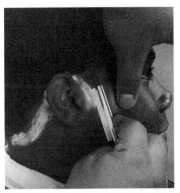

FIGURE 160 | Shave down the side of the neck.

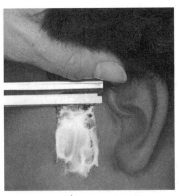

FIGURE 161 | Shave the left sideburn using reverse backhand or backhand stroke.

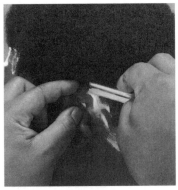

FIGURE 162A | Shave around ear

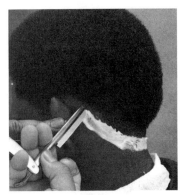

FIGURE 162B | Shave behind the ear to the nape corner.

   e. Shave the side of the neck below the ear, using the backhand stroke with the point of the razor (Figure 162b). Hold the ear away with the fingers of the left hand. If the stroke is done with one continuous movement, a straight line will be formed down the side of the neck.

   f. Shave the nape area with a freehand stroke (Figure 163).

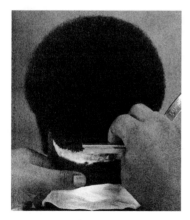

FIGURE 163 | Shave the nape area (optional).

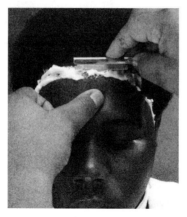

FIGURE 164 | Step 5 (optional): Start at the front hairline and shave in the center.

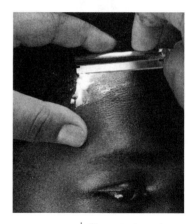

FIGURE 165 | Shave to temple corner.

4 Front hairline:
   a. Start in the center of the front hairline and work toward the corners using a freehand stroke to the client's right side and a backhand stroke to the client's left side (Figure 164).
   b. Follow the natural hairline, shaving the outline through the temporal (crest, horseshoe, etc.) area to the front corner of the sideburns (Figure 165).

▷ procedure no. 6

Fingers-and-Shear Technique

Preparation

1 Conduct client consultation.

2 Drape the client for wet service.

3 Shampoo and towel dry hair.

4 Remove the waterproof cape and replace it with a neckstrip and haircutting chair cloth.

5 Face the client toward the mirror and lock the chair.

Reminder: Maintain uniform moisture throughout the haircutting procedure.

Step 1

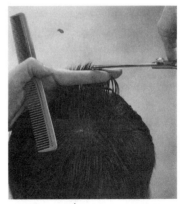

FIGURE 166 | Step 1: Establish guide for top section.

1 Comb the hair down in front, sides, and back. Standing behind the model, take a 1/4- to 1/2-inch parting (depending on the density of the hair) at the forward-most part of the crown.

2 Comb the parting straight up at 90 degrees and hold it between the fingers of the left hand.

3 Bend the parting from right to left to determine at what length the hair will bend (bending point) to lie down smoothly (usually between 2 and 3 inches). When this length has been determined, recomb the parting and, using the fingers of the left hand as a level, cut the hair that extends beyond the fingers (Figure 166). This cut establishes the traveling guide for the top section.

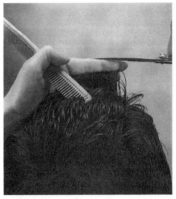

FIGURE 167A | Hold each parting at a 90-degree elevation while working toward the front.

4 Pick up a second parting, retaining the guideline, comb, and cut. (The guideline should be visible and parallel to the top of the fingers.) A rhythm will soon develop: part hair for parting (1); comb hair in front of parting forward (so it doesn't interfere with first parting) (2); comb parting, retaining previous guide (3); and, cut hair that extends past the guideline (4).

5 Complete the top section of hair, moving forward toward the front with each parting and cut. Remember to hold each parting that is to be cut at a 90-degree elevation from where it grows (Figures 167a and 167b).

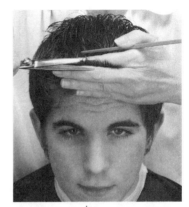

FIGURE 167B | Front view of last 90-degree parting in top section.

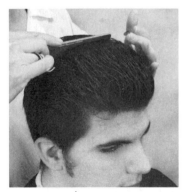

FIGURE 168 | Step 2: Comb the top section back.

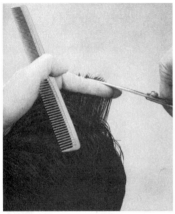

FIGURE 169 | Hold the original guide and 1/2-inch section of hair at the crown.

Step 2

1. Comb the top section back (Figure 168). Move to the client's left side. Starting at the forehead, part off the top section of hair, front to back, with the thumb and middle finger.

2. Hold the original guideline and a 1/2-inch parting at the crown at 90 degrees, and cut (Figure 169). This establishes the guide for the crown and back sections.

3. Work forward, still maintaining a side-standing position. Following the arc and contour of the head, even off any length that does not blend with the traveling guide (Figure 170). If step 1 was performed correctly, no more than 1/4 inch of hair should need to be evened or blended. Step 2 is a checkpoint for your work in the top section (Figure 171).

Step 3

1. Comb the hair forward and move in front of the client (Figure 172). Holding the front hair section

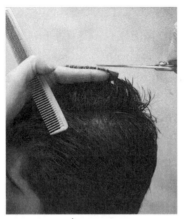

FIGURE 170 | Follow the arc of the head, trimming strands that do not blend with the traveling guide.

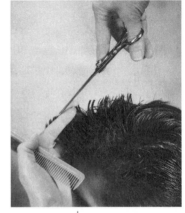

FIGURE 171 | Step 2 is the checkpoint for work in the top section.

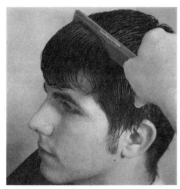

FIGURE 172 | Step 3: Comb the hair forward.

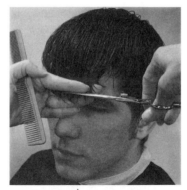

FIGURE 173 | Establish front design line.

between the fingers of the left hand at 0 degrees, begin in the center and cut to the desired length to establish the front design line (Figure 173). Cut right, and then left of the center to the ends of the width of the eyebrows, or to include the temporal area. The front and temporal design line has just been completed and will act as a traveling guide for the temporal area.

Step 4

1. Move behind the client.

2. Beginning on the right side, pick up the front hair of the temporal/crest region. A small amount of the previously cut top hair should be visible.

3. Hold the hair at 90 degrees and cut to the top guide (Figures 174a and 174b).

4. Continue cutting the crest area, working back to the center of the crown area (Figures 175a and 175b). Cut hair only from the temporal region; do not pick up side hair. When approaching the crown area, reposition yourself so as to move toward the client's left, but not as far as the side of the model.

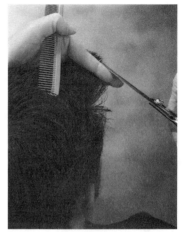

FIGURE 174A | Step 4: Hold front temporal section at 90 degrees and cut to the top guide.

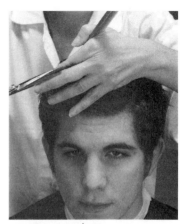

FIGURE 174B | Front view of cutting right temporal section.

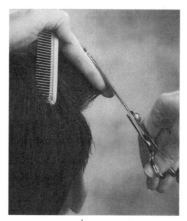

FIGURE 175A | Continue cutting through the crest (temporal) area.

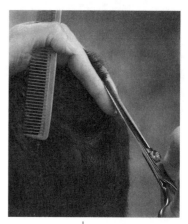

FIGURE 175B | Work back to the center of the crown.

Step 5

1 Repeat the step 4 procedure on the left side of the client's hair. Cuts will be made *from* the top guide through the temporal region, rather than *to* the top guide. If the front design line was cut correctly, the excess hair in the front temporal region should not exceed 1 to 1 1/2 inches. The crown hair from the right and left sides should meet upon completion of step 5 (Figures 176a and 176b).

2 The top, temporal, and crown areas are now cut.

3 Comb the hair for step 6.

Step 6

1 Moving to the right of the client, comb the hair straight down on the sides.

2 Take a 1/4- to 1/2-inch horizontal parting at the hairline, from the top of the ear to the sideburn area, and a diagonal parting of the same thickness from the right temple to the sideburn (Figure 177).

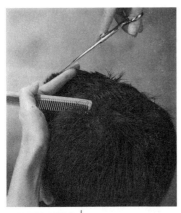

FIGURE 176A | Step 1: Repeat step 4 on left side.

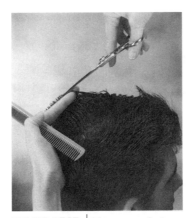

FIGURE 176B | The crown hair from the right and left should meet.

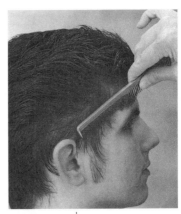

FIGURE 177 | Step 2: Comb down parting from hairline.

3   Comb the remaining hair back or secure it with a hair clip.

4   Cut the design line either around the ears or to cover part of the ears at the desired length (Figure 178). If cutting around the ear, gently bend or slightly tug the ear down out of the way (Figure 179).

5   Move toward the front of the client, facing the temporal and side areas.

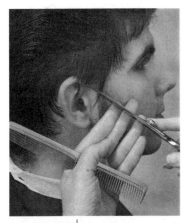

FIGURE 178 | Cut side hair to desired length.

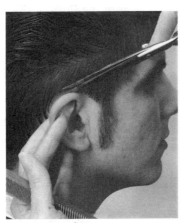

FIGURE 179 | Gently tug the ear down.

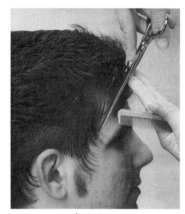

FIGURE 180 | Use the front and side design lines as guides to cut along the natural hairline.

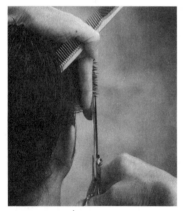

FIGURE 181 | Pick up vertical partings at 90 degrees.

6 Using the front and side design lines (which are acting as guides), cut the hair between these two points at 0 degrees against the skin, cutting along the natural hairline (Figure 180).

7 Holding the hair between the fingers at 0 degrees, check the design line cut.

8 Proceed cutting the remaining side hair section, repeating the partings as the density of the hair requires.

9 Repeat this procedure on the left side, then check the length of the sides in the mirror for evenness.

10 Move behind the client. Pick up the hair in vertical partings, holding it straight out to the side at 90 degrees. The design/guide line should be visible at the tips of the fingers when working on the right side of the client's head (Figure 181).

11 Make a straight, vertical cut from the design/guide line, cutting off any hair that extends past the guide.

12 Continue cutting partings of hair while following the contour of the head until reaching the temporal/crest region (Figures 182a and 182b). The hair lengths should meet and blend. Check the procedure by checking the blend of hair from the side design/guide line to the top section guide.

13 Proceed until all the side hair is cut. Stop at the topmost point behind the ear. Repeat for the left side. You may be positioned facing the client in order to work from the design/guide line up when blending the hair, or you may prefer to remain behind the client.

14 The front, top, temporal, crown, and side areas are now cut.

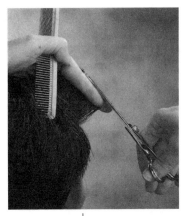

FIGURE 182A | Follow the contour of the head.

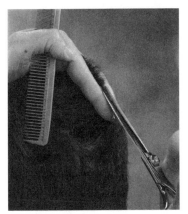

FIGURE 182B | Blend the side hair to the crest.

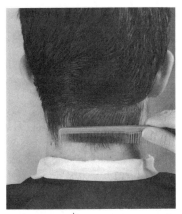

FIGURE 183 | Step 7: Section off a parting from the nape.

Step 7

1. Move behind the client. Section off a 1/4- to 1/2-inch horizontal parting at the nape of the neck (Figure 183). Secure excess hair with a clip if necessary.

2. Starting in the center of the nape, cut the hair to the desired length; cut left and then right, to the corners of the nape area (Figure 184). Check the design line cut.

3. Move to the client's right side. Part off a 1/4- to 1/2-inch section along the hairline. Cut hair in a downward direction from the side design line guide to right nape corner (Figure 185).

4. Comb and check the cut. Repeat for the left side. A backhand shear cutting position is required to cut downward on the client's left side (Figure 186).

5. Part off a subsequent parting and comb hair down. Holding the design/guide line and parting between the fingers, cut hair at 0 degrees (Figure 187). Complete 0-degree cutting at the nape and behind-the-ear areas as density requires (Figure 188).

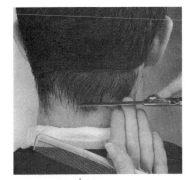

FIGURE 184 | Begin back design line at center of nape; cut to corners.

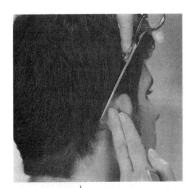

FIGURE 185 | Cut from side guide to nape corner along hairline.

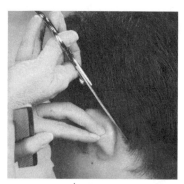

FIGURE 186 | Repeat step 7 on the left side.

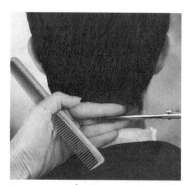

FIGURE 187 | Cut subsequent nape partings at 0 degrees.

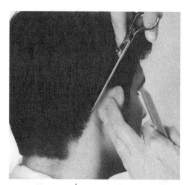

FIGURE 188 | Complete 0-degree cutting behind the ears to the nape.

6   Pick up the hair in vertical partings at 90 degrees; blend through the back section up to meet the guides in the crown and crest areas (Figures 189 and 190).

7   Proceed until the entire back section is cut and sides are blended to the back (Figure 191).

8   Check the entire haircut by combing the hair up in 90-degree sections, making sure that the hair blends from one section to another.

9   Perform a neck shave and shave outline areas as desired.

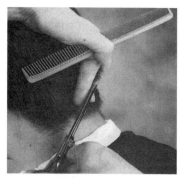

FIGURE 189 | Pick up vertical parting at 90 degrees and blend through back section.

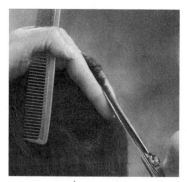

FIGURE 190 | Blend back section to meet crown and crest areas.

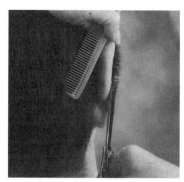

FIGURE 191 | Blend sides to the back.

Step 8

1. Dry the client's hair in a free-form style. This method requires the barber to move the dryer briskly from side to side while drying the hair. Begin at the nape, using a brush or comb in the left hand to hold midsection hair out of the way while drying the underneath hair first. The nozzle of the dryer should be pointing downward, 6 to 10 inches away from the hair. As the hair dries, check the cut for blending qualities. Proceed to dry the sides and top.

2. Brush the hair into place using a directional nozzle, if needed.

3. Use a trimmer (outliner) to clean up sideburns, sides (in around-the-ear styles), and nape (Figures 192, 193, and 194). Check the behind-the-ear area for any difference in hair length or design. Complete finish work by performing a neck shave after outlining the bottom of the sideburn and around-the-ear areas with a razor.

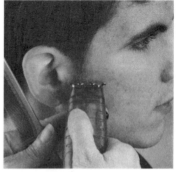

FIGURE 192 | Step 8: Trim the sideburns.

4. Recomb the hair into the finished style (Figure 195).

5. Consult with the client regarding the use of a styling aid.

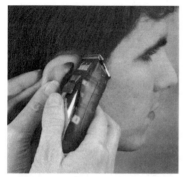

FIGURE 193 | Trim around the ears.

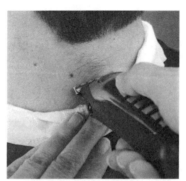

FIGURE 194 | Trim and clean up the nape.

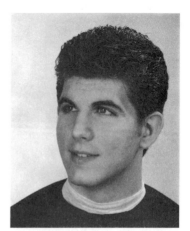

FIGURE 195 | Finished style.

6   The haircut and style are now complete. Dust or vacuum stray hairs, making sure none remain on the client's face or neck.

▷ procedure no. 7

Alternative Fingers-and-Shear Technique

Some barbers prefer to begin fingers-and-shear cutting in the front section or with a side part established in the hair.

Preparation

1   Conduct client consultation.

2   Drape the client for wet service.

3   Shampoo and towel dry hair.

4   Remove the waterproof cape and replace it with a neckstrip and haircutting chair cloth.

5   Face the client toward the mirror and lock the chair.

Reminder: Maintain uniform moisture throughout the haircutting procedure.

Step 1

Comb client's hair into desired style with a side part. Start at the front hairline and project a parting of hair to 90 degrees. Cut to desired length and use as a traveling guide to cut back toward the crown (Figure 196).

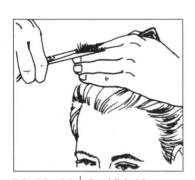

FIGURE 196 | Establish 90-degree guide in front top section.

Step 2

Pick up hair from the front temporal/crest area using the same procedure as in step 1 to cut back toward the crown (Figure 197).

Continue cutting all around the crest area through to the left side; or, stop at the center of the crown and repeat procedure on the left side, working from the front to the crown. Continue with steps 6–8 of Procedure No. 13.

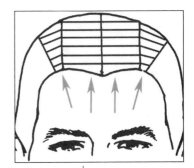

FIGURE 197 | Diagram for alternate fingers-and-shear technique.

▷ procedure no. 8

Shear-over-Comb Technique

Preparation

1 Conduct client consultation.

2 Drape the client for wet service.

3 Shampoo and towel dry hair. Blow-dry hair if dry cutting is preferred.

4 Remove the waterproof cape and replace it with a neckstrip and haircutting chair cloth.

5 Face the client toward the mirror and lock the chair (Figure 198a).

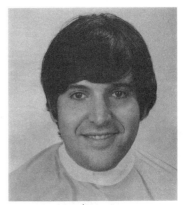

FIGURE 198A | Before shear-over-comb technique.

Step 1

Comb the hair. Start cutting in the nape area, trimming hair to the desired length and thickness up to the occipital (Figure 198b).

Step 2

Move to right side and begin shear-over-comb cutting from the sideburn hairline into the side section (Figure 199).

Step 3

Continue technique over and behind the right ear (Figure 200).

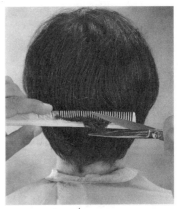

FIGURE 198B | Start in nape area and cut to the occipital.

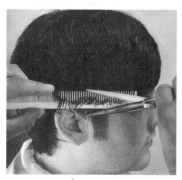

FIGURE 199 | Cut from the sideburn into side section.

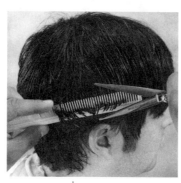

FIGURE 200 | Continue cutting over and behind the ear.

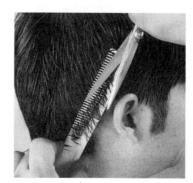

FIGURE 201 | Use a diagonal comb position from side to nape corner.

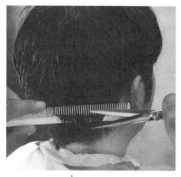

FIGURE 202 | Blend hair into back section.

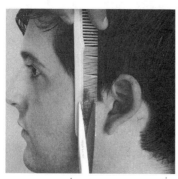

FIGURE 203 | Repeat sideburn and side section cutting on left side.

Step 4

Using a diagonal comb position, blend the hair behind the ear to the hair at the right corner of the nape along the hairline (Figure 201).

Step 5

Blend hair at the side of the neck into the back section (Figure 202).

Step 6

Move to left side and repeat shear-over-comb cutting from the sideburn hairline into the side section (Figure 203).

Step 7

Continue technique over and in back of the left ear.

Step 8

Using a diagonal comb position, blend the hair behind the ear to the hair at the left corner of the nape along the hairline (Figure 204).

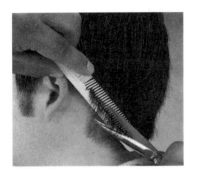

FIGURE 204 | Blend hair behind ear to left nape corner.

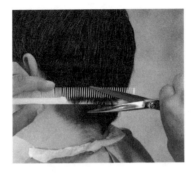

FIGURE 205 | Blend hair at side of neck into back section.

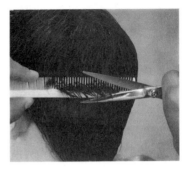

FIGURE 206 | Blend hair from occipital to crown.

Step 9

Blend hair at the side of the neck into the back section (Figure 205).

Step 10

Blend hair from the occipital to the crown (Figure 206).

Step 11

Blend hair from the crown through the right and left crest areas into the top section (Figure 207). Trim front section to an appropriate length for blending with the top and crest.

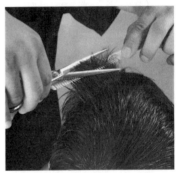

FIGURE 207 | Blend hair from crown through crest and top areas.

Step 12

Outline sideburns, around the ear, and behind-the-ear areas with shears, followed by the trimmer (Figure 208). Finish the haircut with a neck and/or outline shave as the client desires. Also consult with the client regarding the use of a styling aid. Style the hair as desired. The haircut and style are now complete (Figure 209). Dust or vacuum any stray hairs on the client's face or neck.

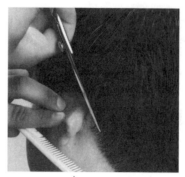

FIGURE 208 | Outline with shears, followed by the trimmer.

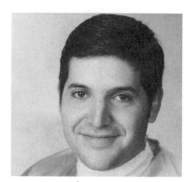

FIGURE 209 | Finished shear-over-comb cut.

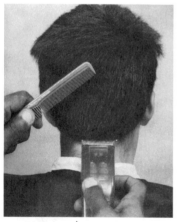

FIGURE 210A | Step 1: Start in the nape area.

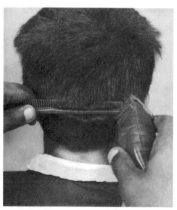

FIGURE 210B | Cut to the occipital.

▷ procedure no. 9

Freehand and Clipper-over-Comb Technique with Straight Hair

Preparation

1. Conduct client consultation.

2. Drape the client for wet service.

3. Shampoo and towel dry hair. Blow-dry hair if dry cutting is preferred.

4. Remove the waterproof cape and replace it with a neckstrip and haircutting chair cloth.

5. Face client toward the mirror and lock the chair.

Step 1

Comb the hair. Start in nape area and freehand taper the first inch or so of hair. Proceed with clipper-over-comb cutting to the occipital and lower crown areas (Figures 210a and 210b).

Step 2

Move to right side and establish the length of the sideburn (Figure 211a). Begin clipper-over-comb cutting from the sideburn hairline into the side section (Figure 211b).

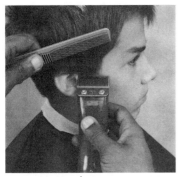

FIGURE 211A | Step 2: Establish the length of the sideburn.

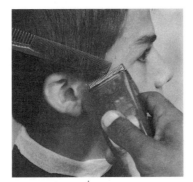

FIGURE 211B | Blend from the sideburn into the side section.

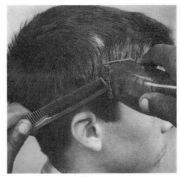

FIGURE 212A | Step 3: Blend hair above the right ear.

Step 3

Continue technique above and in back of the right ear (Figures 212a and 212b).

Step 4

Using a diagonal comb position, blend the hair behind the ear to the hair at the right corner of the nape along the hairline (Figure 213a).

Step 5

Blend hair on the right side of the neck into the back section (Figure 213b).

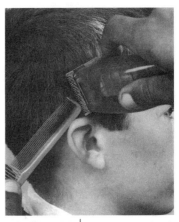

FIGURE 212B | Blend hair in back of right ear.

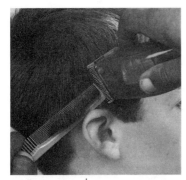

FIGURE 213A | Step 4: Position comb diagonally to blend behind the ear.

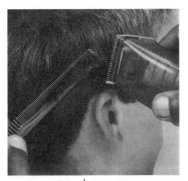

FIGURE 213B | Blend to back section.

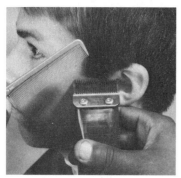

FIGURE 214 | Step 6: Establish sideburn length and cut side section.

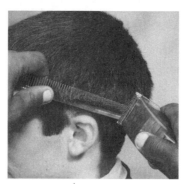

FIGURE 215 | Step 7: Blend around the ear.

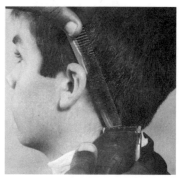

FIGURE 216 | Step 8: Blend sides to left nape corner.

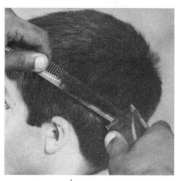

FIGURE 217 | Steps 5 through 9: Blend sides to back section.

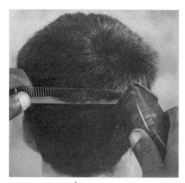

FIGURE 218 | Step 10: Blend from occipital to crown.

Step 6

Move to left side, establish sideburn length and begin clipper-over-comb, cutting into the side section (Figure 214).

Step 7

Continue technique above and in back of the left ear (Figure 215).

Step 8

Using a diagonal comb position, blend the hair behind the ear to the hair at the left corner of the nape along the hairline (Figure 216).

Step 9

Blend hair at the side of the neck into the back section (Figure 217).

Step 10

Blend hair from the occipital to the crown (Figure 218).

Step 11

Blend hair from the crown through the right and left crest areas to meet the side sections. (Figure 219). Trim top section using

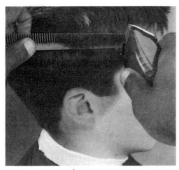

FIGURE 219 | Step 11: Blend crest and side.

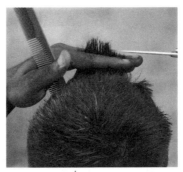

FIGURE 220 | Trim top section.

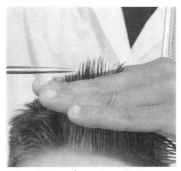

FIGURE 221 | Check for evenness and blending.

fingers-and-shear method to achieve the desired length (Figure 220). Check blending and fine-tune using fingers-and-shear method (Figure 221).

Step 12

Outline sideburns, around the ear, back of the ear areas, and nape with shears and then trimmer. Complete finish work by performing a neck shave after outlining the bottom of the sideburn and around-the-ear areas with a razor. Consult with the client regarding the use of a styling aid, then style the hair as desired. The haircut and style is now complete (Figure 222). Dust or vacuum any stray hairs from the client's face or neck.

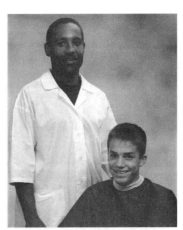

FIGURE 222 | Finished style.

▷ procedure no. 10

Freehand and Clipper-over-Comb Technique with Tightly Curled Hair

1. Conduct client consultation.

2. Drape the client for wet service.

3. Shampoo and towel dry hair. Blow-dry hair if dry cutting is preferred.

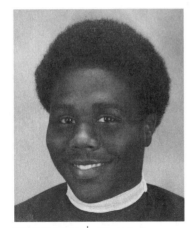

FIGURE 223A | Client before haircut.

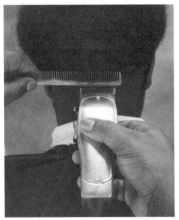

FIGURE 223B | Step 1: Clipper-over-comb taper (or freehand taper) nape to occipital.

4 Remove the waterproof cape and replace it with a neckstrip and haircutting chair cloth.

5 Face client toward the mirror and lock the chair (Figure 223a).

Step 1

Comb or pick the hair out. Start in nape area and freehand taper or clipper-over-comb taper the first inch or so of hair (Figure 223b). If hair density allows, proceed with clipper-over-comb cutting to the occipital area. If the hair is thick, freehand clipper cut to the occipital area.

Step 2

Move to right side and use freehand or clipper-over-comb to cut and blend from the sideburn hairline up to the crest (Figure 224).

Step 3

Continue technique above and in back of the right ear (Figure 225).

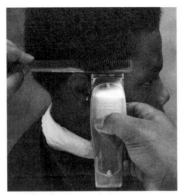

FIGURE 224 | Step 2: Cut and blend to the crest.

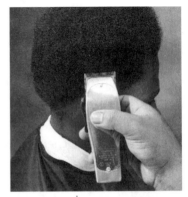

FIGURE 225 | Step 3: Blend above and in back of ear.

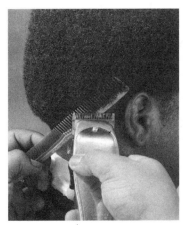

FIGURE 226 | Step 4: Blend from side to nape corner.

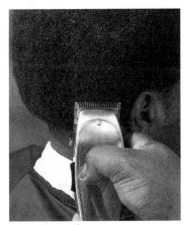

FIGURE 227 | Step 5: Blend into back section.

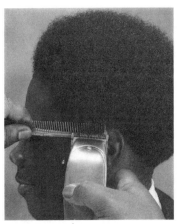

FIGURE 228 | Step 6: Cut from sideburn to crest.

Step 4

Using a diagonal comb position, blend the hair behind the ear to the hair at the right corner of the nape along the hairline; or, freehand the entire section (Figure 226).

Step 5

Blend hair at the side of the neck into the back section (Figure 227).

Step 6

Move to left side and begin freehand or clipper-over-comb cutting from the sideburn hairline to the crest (Figure 228).

Step 7

Continue technique above and in back of the left ear (Figure 229).

Step 8

Using a diagonal comb or freehand position, blend the hair behind the ear to the hair at the left corner of the nape along the hairline (Figure 230).

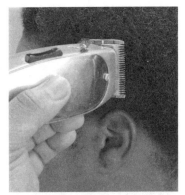

FIGURE 229 | Step 7: Cut above and in back of left ear.

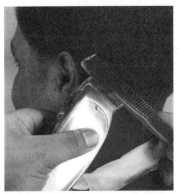

FIGURE 230 | Step 8: Blend behind ear to nape corner.

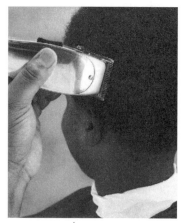

FIGURE 231 | Step 9: Blend hair into back section.

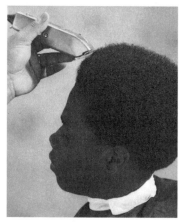

FIGURE 232 | Step 10: Establish guide in front center section, cut back to crown.

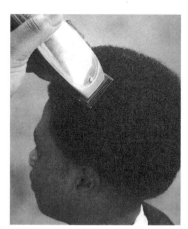

FIGURE 233 | Step 11: Blend crest to top guide.

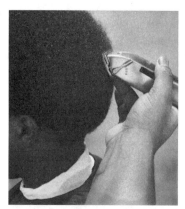

FIGURE 234 | Step 12: Blend occipital area to crest. Check blending to top section.

Step 9

Blend hair at the side of the neck into the back section (Figure 231).

Step 10

Establish guide in front center of top section and cut back to crown area (Figure 232).

Step 11

Blend crest to top guide around the entire head (Figure 233).

Step 12

Blend occipital area to crest, then check the blend to the top section (Figure 234).

Step 13

Comb or pick hair out. Fine-tune with shears (Figure 235).

Step 14

Outline sideburns, around the ear, and back of the ear areas with clippers or trimmers. Consult with the client regarding the use of a styling aid and style the hair as desired. The haircut and style portion of the service is now complete. Finish with the neck and outline shaving procedures. Dust or vacuum stray hairs from the client's face and neck.

▷ procedure no. 11

Razor Cutting

1. Conduct client consultation.
2. Drape the client for wet service.
3. Shampoo and towel dry hair.
4. Remove the waterproof cape and replace it with a neckstrip and haircutting chair cloth.
5. Face client toward the mirror and lock the chair.

Step 1

Section the hair into four sections from crown to nape, crown to front, and crest to sides. Subdivide the back section into three subsections (Figure 236).

Step 2

Begin in the center section just below the crown. Taper the hair using the razor rotation technique, one strip at a time in a downward direction to the hairline. Blend each new cut with the hair previously trimmed. Use short, even razor strokes to avoid ridges, lines, or any appearance of unevenness (Figure 237).

Step 3

Comb the hair downward from the top right side toward the left midsection in the back. Lightly taper from right to left in the

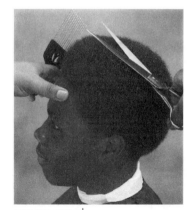

FIGURE 235 | Step 13: Fine-tune with shears.

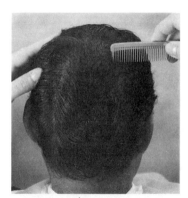

FIGURE 236 | Step 1: Sectioning for razor cut.

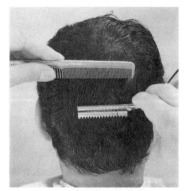

FIGURE 237 | Step 2: Begin razor rotation.

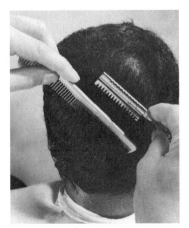

FIGURE 238 | Step 3: Lightly taper from top right to left midsection.

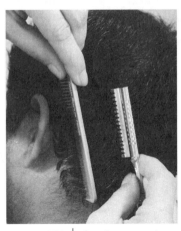

FIGURE 239 | Continue tapering through lower left section.

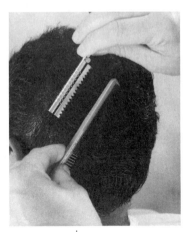

FIGURE 240 | Step 4: Repeat step 3, working from left to right.

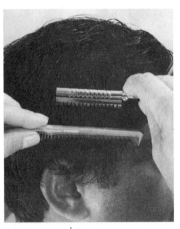

FIGURE 241 | Step 5: Taper from the crest to the hairline.

top section (Figure 238). Taper the lower section to blend with the nape hair (Figure 239).

Step 4

Comb the hair downward from the top left side toward the right. Repeat the procedure used in Step 3 (Figure 240).

Step 5

Comb side hair downward and subdivide it into three vertical partings. Begin tapering about 3/4 of an inch from the crest. Taper downward through the three sections to the hairline (Figure 241). Comb the hair toward the back and taper lightly in that direction, then blend with the back section (Figure 242). Comb the hair forward and taper lightly toward the face, trimming the perimeter (design) line as needed (Figure 243).

Step 6

Repeat step 5 procedures on left side of head (Figure 244).

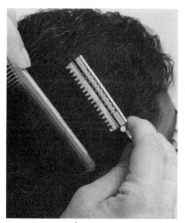

FIGURE 242 | Lightly taper side to blend with back section.

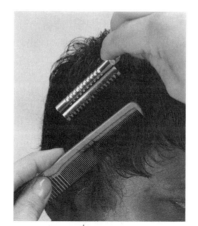

FIGURE 243 | Lightly taper toward the face. Trim design line as needed.

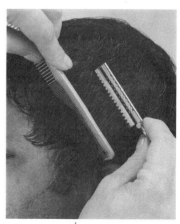

FIGURE 244 | Step 6: Repeat step 5 procedures on left side.

Step 7

Comb top hair forward with even distribution over the head form (Figure 245).

Start tapering, just forward of the crown, in the top section (Figure 246). Work toward the forehead on the right side. Repeat on the left side and then taper the center section. Make sure to blend all three sections. Hold the front section at 0 degrees and trim using the freehand slicing technique (Figure 247).

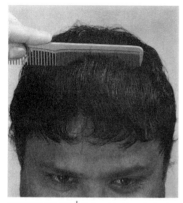

FIGURE 245 | Step 7: Comb hair forward with even distribution.

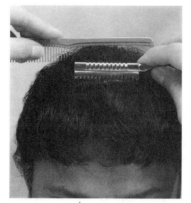

FIGURE 246 | Start tapering in top section.

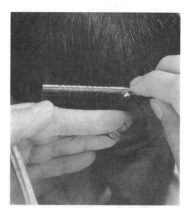

FIGURE 247 | Trim front length using freehand slicing movement.

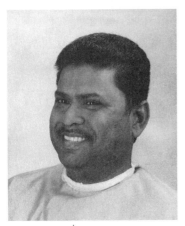

FIGURE 248 | Finished cut and style.

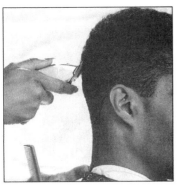

FIGURE 249 | Start at center of nape cutting to just below occipital.

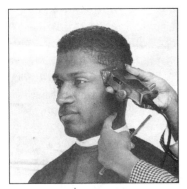

FIGURE 250 | Cut the side section to the crest.

Step 8

Comb through the cut, redistributing the sections in a variety of directions to check for blending and evenness. Consult with the client regarding a neck shave, outline shaving, and the use of styling aids. Style the hair as desired. The haircut and style are now complete (Figure 248). Dust or vacuum stray hairs, making sure none remain on the client's face or neck.

▷ procedure no. 12

Fade Cut

The standard characteristics that apply to the many variations of fade cuts today include a close, tight cut at the sides and back, blending at the occipital and crest areas, and a customized design at the temples and front sections. To facilitate blending, the clipper blades are opened or closed based on the hair's density and curl pattern.

Reminder: Cutting against the grain achieves a closer cut than cutting with the grain. The following procedure offers one method to achieve a close fade cut. Be guided by the desires of your client for technique and fade style variations.

Step 1

Set the clipper blade in the closed position to achieve a close cut. Start at the center of the nape, cutting to just below the occipital (Figure 249). Cut the sections right and left of center.

Step 2

Move to the right side (or left, depending on preference) and cut from the hairline to the top, middle, or bottom of the crest area as desired by the client (Figure 250). Cut around the ear and into the previously cut back section, cutting up and/or across as the growth pattern allows. Complete cutting the left side in the same manner.

Step 3

When the back and sides are completed, open the clipper blades (one-quarter of the way for fine hair; almost one-half for thick hair) to begin blending a 1/4-inch horizontal section at the point you stopped cutting at the crest. Continue cutting only the 1/4-inch section from the right side, across the back, and into the left side area. *Option:* You may choose to stop at the center back and cut *from* the left side to the center back. Repeat as required to completely blend that section of the crest area around the entire head.

Step 4

Open the blade another quarter and repeat the procedure in step 3, cutting another 1/4-inch section above the one previously cut. Repeat a third time.

Step 5

Place a #1 guard on the clipper blades and position the lever halfway open. The guard will facilitate blending into the longer lengths of the top section. When complete, remove the guard and use a clipper-over-comb technique all around the head for final blending.

Step 6

Layer the top section uniformly and blend with previously cut hair in the crest areas. Finish with the trimmer and/or outline shave to define the hairline (Figure 251).

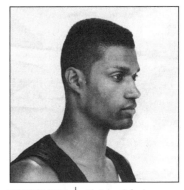

FIGURE 251 | Finished fade style.

▷ procedure no. 13

Head Shaving

The shaved head is one of today's current fashion trends that is chosen by many men regardless of the density or growth pattern

■ TECH TERM

An *abrasion* is a scrape of the skin, an irritation, or a wearing off of the skin's surface. A *lesion* is a structural change in the tissues caused by injury or disease.

of their hair. A head shave should be performed with a changeable-blade or conventional straight razor.

The following is one method used to perform a head shave.

Step 1

Examine the scalp for any abrasions, primary or secondary lesions, or scalp disorders.

Step 2

Remove excess hair length with the clippers. Use a balding clipper blade if available. Shampoo the remaining hair and reexamine the scalp.

Step 3

Apply shaving cream or gel and lather. Next, apply two or three steam towel treatments to soften the remaining hair.

Step 4

Start at the back and use a freehand stroke to shave with the grain of the hair from the crown to the nape. Use the opposite hand to stretch the skin taut as needed for each area to be shaved. Follow the curve of the head, taking short strokes with the first half of the blade from its point to midsection.

Step 5

Move in front of the client and tip his head forward slightly. Continue shaving from the crown to the front hairline, reapplying lathering agent as needed.

NOTE: Keep the skin moist to facilitate shaving.

Step 6

When the top section is completed, work down the sides. Just below the crest, hold the ear out of the way with the left hand, finish shaving the side, and carefully shave in front of and around the ears.

Step 7

Upon completion of the head shave, check for any missed areas. Remove remaining lather with a warm towel, apply witch hazel or toner, and follow with a cool towel application for two to three minutes.

INTRODUCTION TO MEN'S HAIRSTYLING

Hairstyling is the art of arranging the hair into an appropriate style following a haircut or shampoo. Today, many haircuts require minimal hairstyling techniques due to the quality of the cuts and the availability of effective styling aids such as gels, mousses, and styling sprays. Other haircuts require more styling attention, such as blow-drying or picking the style into place. In some cases, even finger-waving techniques are used to create the final style, so it is important that barbers are versatile in all the techniques.

Blow-Dry Styling

Blow-dry styling—the technique of drying and styling damp hair in one operation—has revolutionized the hair care industry. Though most men may not wish to do more than to comb the hair into place, the use of a blow-dryer offers some options for speed-drying and special-effects styling.

The main parts of a blow-dryer are the handle, nozzle, fan, heating element, speed/heat and cooling buttons. The nozzle is a directional feature that helps to direct the airstream to a more concentrated area. A diffuser attachment disperses the airflow to a larger area, creating a softer stream while still allowing the heat for drying purposes (Figure 252).

The implements most often used to style men's hair with a blow-dryer are combs, picks, and a variety of brushes. Some

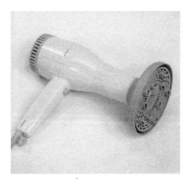

FIGURE 252 | Blow-dryer and diffuser.

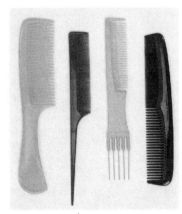

FIGURE 253 | Combs.

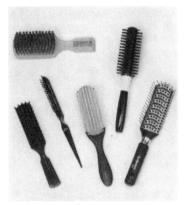

FIGURE 254 | Brushes.

barbers prefer a narrow brush with wire or hard plastic bristles. Others prefer vent or grooming brushes. In most cases, the texture of the hair and the desired effect will dictate the type of implement to use (Figures 253 and 254).

Three general blow-drying techniques are used in men's hairstyling: free-form, stylized, and diffused.

Blow-Drying Techniques

Free-form blow-drying is a quick, easy method of drying the client's hair. This technique can build fullness into the style while allowing the hair to fall into the natural lines of the cut (Figures 255 through 257). Some barbers choose this method for the following reasons:

- It shows the client the ease with which the style can be duplicated.

- It demonstrates the quality of the haircut as the hair falls into place.

- The blow-drying service is accelerated.

- It allows the barber to check the accuracy of the work as the hair falls into place.

Stylized blow-drying creates a more styled appearance because each section is dried in a definite direction with the aid of a comb or brush. It may be performed with or without styling products applied to damp hair (Figures 258, 259a, and 259b).

Diffused drying is used when the client desires to maintain the natural wave pattern of the hair, as opposed to temporarily straightening it with the blow-dryer and brush. Diffused drying is an effective option to use when arranging or picking out very curly hair textures, manipulating sculpting and styling products, or employing scrunching techniques (Figures 260 through 262).

Building Volume

Occasionally extra volume is needed in the crown, crest, or top (apex) areas of a style to create a more proportionate look. To build volume and/or to create an even contour throughout the hairstyle, use the dryer and brush in the following manner:

1. Lift the hair with a brush, bending the section as the blow-dryer is directed at the base of the section and followed through to the ends. Avoid burning the scalp.

2. Follow the same procedure to build fullness on the sides. Use horizontal partings if the hair is to be styled down on the sides and vertical or diagonal partings if the hair will be brushed back.

▷ procedure no. 14

Blow-Drying Techniques

Free-Form Blow-Drying

1   Hold the blow-dryer in the dominant hand. The dryer should be held 6 to 10 inches from the area being dried, at an angle with the nozzle pointing downward on the hair, and should be moved briskly from side to side as it dries the hair.

2   Beginning at the nape area, hold the hair above the hairline out of the way with a brush or comb in the opposite hand (Figure 255). As the hair underneath is dried, the brush or comb releases the next layered section for drying. Comb or brush the hair down after each section is dried.

3   Dry the sides in the same manner (Figure 256).

4   The top should be dried loosely and then brushed in to the desired style, followed by the dryer (Figure 257).

5   Apply different styling aids such as mousses, gels, and hair sprays to compare and contrast the effects.

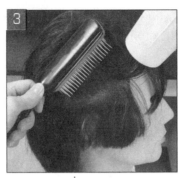

FIGURE 255 | Free-form blow-drying nape and back sections.

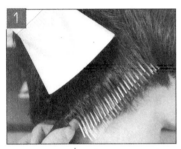

FIGURE 256 | Drying the side section.

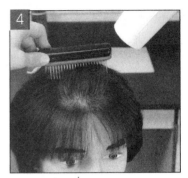

FIGURE 257 | Drying the front section.

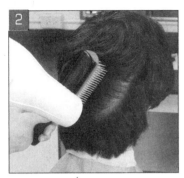

FIGURE 258 | Follow the brush with concentrated heat from the dryer.

Stylized Blow-Drying

1   Begin in the back section and lift a section of hair with the comb or brush. While combing or brushing through the parting, follow the movement with the dryer to apply a concentrated stream of heated air to the section. Repeat the process until the hair is dry in that section and continue the process with subsequent partings or sections of hair (Figure 258).

2   Dry the sides in the same manner.

3   To create lift or direction in the top section, work from the natural part, parting off a section with the comb or brush. Elevate for desired fullness and follow with the blow-dryer.

4   To create a definite direction in the front section, the comb or brush can be used on top of a section of hair along the hairline. Insert the comb/brush about 1 1/2 inches from the hairline, first drawing the comb/brush a little to the back and then toward the hairline in one motion. This will create a ridge or bend in the hair that will "set it" in a different direction (Figure 259a). Lift the hair for volume (Figure 259b). Adjust the blow-dryer to hot and direct the hot air back and forth until a soft ridge has been

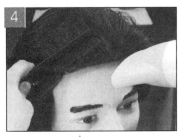

FIGURE 259A | Create a ridge or bend in the hair with the comb.

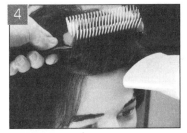

FIGURE 259B | Lift the hair for volume.

formed. Repeat, following these instructions, for subsequent sections in the top and crest areas.

5 Apply a suitable styling aid to finish the styling service.

Diffused Drying

1 Pick the hair out into the basic shape of the desired style (Figure 260).

2 Begin drying in the back section, working toward the crown and sides. Gently pick the hair out as the dryer is moved from section to section (Figure 261).

3 Dry the sides in the same manner.

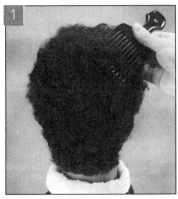

FIGURE 260 | Pick out the hair.

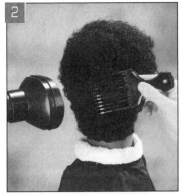

FIGURE 261 | Begin drying in the back section.

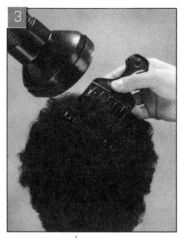

FIGURE 262 | Dry top section.

4   Dry the top section forward from the crown, picking the hair out as each area is dried (Figure 262).

5   Apply a suitable styling aid to complete the styling service.

Braids and Locks

The techniques associated with styling the hair into braids and locks is a form of *natural hair care* that originated in Africa thousands of years ago. Natural hair care has gained such popularity that an entirely new division of the hair care industry has developed. As a recognized professional segment of our industry, natural hair care is an active and exciting division that is currently involved in education, licensing, and legislative changes to meet the needs of its educators, practitioners, and clients.

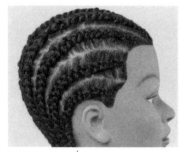

FIGURE 263 | Cornrows.

Braids

Although many variations of braids and braiding styles are popular, *on-the-scalp cornrows* is one of the most popular styles chosen by men today (Figure 263). If the client has very short hair, you will be working close to the scalp across the curves of the head. The braid may begin at the nape, top, or sides depending on the desired finished result.

▷ procedure no. 15

Creating Cornrows

Figures 264 through 267 illustrate the underhand braiding method used to create cornrows.

1   Apply and massage essential oil to the scalp (Figure 264). Determine the correct size and direction of the cornrow base. Create two parallel partings to form a neat row for the cornrow base (Figure 265).

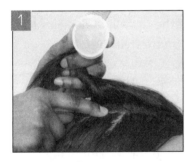

FIGURE 264 | Massage essential oil through hair.

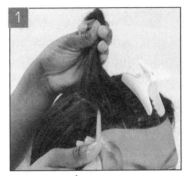

FIGURE 265 | Part out a panel.

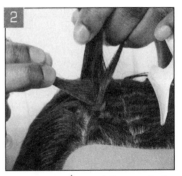

FIGURE 266 | Pass left strand of hair under center strand.

2   Divide the parting into three strands. Place fingers close to the base and cross the left strand under the center strand (Figure 266).

3   Cross the right strand under the center strand (Figure 267).

4   With each crossing under, pick up hair from the base of the panel and add it to the outer strand before crossing it under the center strand (Figures 268 and 269).

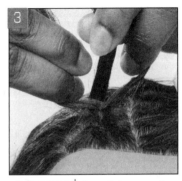

FIGURE 267 | Pass right strand under center strand.

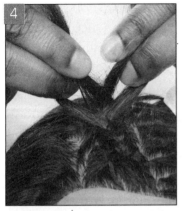

FIGURE 268 | Add hair to left outer strand.

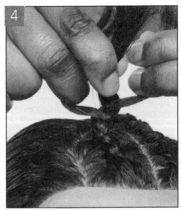

FIGURE 269 | Add hair to right outer strand.

5   Braid subsequent panels in the same manner. Finish with oil sheen or an appropriate styling aid for a finished look.

Locks

Locks, also known as dreadlocks, are created from natural textured hair that is intertwined together to form a single network of hair. Hairlocking is the process that occurs when coily hair is allowed to develop in its natural state without the use of combs, heat, or chemicals. The more coil revolutions within a single strand, the faster the hair will coil and lock.

Cultivated locks are those that are intentionally guided through the natural process of locking. There are several ways to cultivate locks, such as twisting, braiding, and wrapping. The preferred and most effective technique is palm or finger rolling, depending on the length of the hair.

When consulting with the client who is considering locks, it is important to stress the following:

- Once locked, the locks can be removed only by cutting them off.

- The hair locks in progressive stages that can take from six months to a year to complete.

- General maintenance includes regular shop visits for cleaning, conditioning, and rerolling. Once the hair locks into compacted coils, it may be shampooed regularly and managed with a non-petroleum-based oil. Heavy oils should be avoided.

Two basic methods for locking men's hair, which is traditionally shorter at the beginning of the locking process, are the comb technique and the palm- or finger-rolling method. The procedures are as follows:

- *Comb technique.* This method is particularly effective during the early stages of locking and involves placing the comb at the base of the scalp and spiraling the hair into a curl with a rotating motion. With each revolution, the comb moves down along the strand until it reaches the end of the hair shaft.

- *Palm or finger rolling.* This method takes advantage of the hair's natural tendency and ability to coil. Rolling begins with shampooed and conditioned hair. Next, part the hair in horizontal rows from the nape to the front hairline and divide the rows into equal subsections. Apply gel to the first subsection to be rolled. Begin rolling at the nape by using the index finger and thumb to pinch the hair near the scalp; then twist the strands in one full clockwise revolution. Use the fingers or palms to repeat the clockwise revolutions down the entire strand (Figure 270). Maintain a constant degree of moisture by spraying with water as needed. Once all the hair has been rolled, place the client under a hood dryer set on low heat. When the hair is completely dry, apply a light oil to add sheen to the hair.

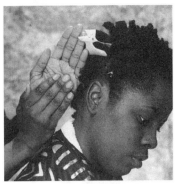

FIGURE 270 | Palm rolling.

Finger Waving Men's Hair

Finger waving is the technique of creating hairstyles with the aid of the fingers, comb, waving or styling lotion or gel, hairpins or clips, and a styling hair net. The best results in developing soft, natural waves are obtained in hair that has a natural or permanent wave.

Finger waves are usually performed with styling lotion and a comb. The styling lotion makes the hair pliable and keeps it in place while creating the waves. As with other products, the styling lotion or gel should be chosen based on the texture and condition of the client's hair. A good styling lotion is harmless to the hair and should not flake after drying. Hard rubber combs with both fine and coarse teeth are recommended for the finger-waving procedure.

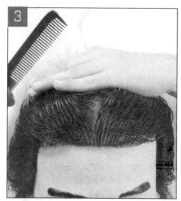

FIGURE 271 | Locate the natural part line.

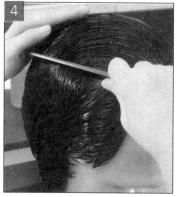

FIGURE 272 | Shape top section with a circular movement.

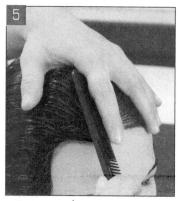

FIGURE 273 | Flatten comb to hold ridge in place.

▷ procedure no. 16

Finger Waving

The finger wave may be started on either side of the head. In this presentation, the work begins on the top right side of the mannequin head.

1. The mannequin should be freshly shampooed and left damp.

2. Comb the hair and arrange it into the basic shape of the desired style. Apply styling lotion and distribute throughout the hair with the comb. Avoid using excessive amounts of styling lotion.

3. Locate the direction of the natural part line by combing the hair away from the face, then pushing it forward with the palm of the hand (Figure 271).

4. Shape the top section using a circular movement starting at the front hairline and work toward the back until the crown has been reached (Figure 272).

5. Place the index finger of the left hand directly above the position for the first ridge. With the teeth of the comb pointing slightly upward, the comb is inserted directly under the index finger. Draw the comb forward about 1 inch along the fingertip. With the teeth still inserted in the ridge, flatten the comb against the head to hold the ridge in place (Figure 273).

6. Remove the left hand from the head and place the middle finger above the ridge and the index finger on the teeth of the comb. Emphasize the ridge by closing the two fingers with pressure (Figure 274).

7. Without removing the comb, turn the teeth down and comb the hair in a right semicircular motion to form a dip in the hollow part of the wave (Figure 275). This

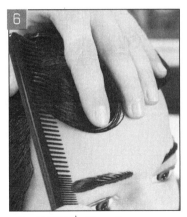

FIGURE 274 | Close fingers to emphasize the ridge.

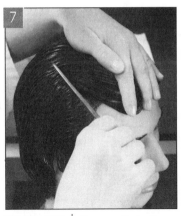

FIGURE 275 | Form a dip in the wave.

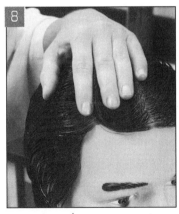

FIGURE 276 | Form a second ridge.

procedure is followed section by section until the crown area has been reached. The ridge and wave of each section should match evenly without showing separations in the ridge and hollow part of the wave.

8   Form the second ridge at the front of the crown area (Figure 276). The movements are the reverse of those followed in forming the first ridge. The comb is drawn back from the fingertip to direct the formation of the second ridge. All movements are followed in a reverse pattern until the hairline is reached and the second ridge is completed (Figure 277).

NOTE: If an additional ridge is required, the movements are the same as for the first ridge.

9   Place a net over the hair and set under hairdryer.

NOTE: Protect the client's forehead and ears with cotton or gauze. Allow the hair to dry thoroughly.

10   Remove the hair net and comb the hair into natural waves.

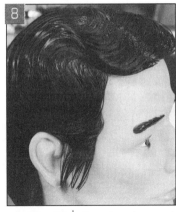

FIGURE 277 | Completed second ridge.

Shadow Waving

Shadow waving is recommended for the sides and sometimes the back of the head form. The wave is made in exactly the same manner as in finger waving, except that the ridges are kept low.

Finger-Waving Guidelines

- Avoid using excessive amounts of styling lotion.
- Locate the natural wave in the hair before beginning the finger wave.
- To emphasize the ridges of a finger wave, press and close the fingers, holding the ridge against the head with pressure.
- To create a longer-lasting finger wave, mold the waves in the direction of the natural hair growth.
- Make sure the hair is thoroughly dried before combing out.
- Use a net to protect the setting pattern while the hair is being dried.

Safety Precautions for Haircutting and Styling

- Use all tools and implements in a safe manner.
- Properly sanitize and store tools and implements.
- Avoid applying dryer heat in one place on the head for too long.
- Keep metal combs away from the scalp when using heat.
- Keep work area clean and sanitized.

FINAL THOUGHTS

In this book we have covered the fundamentals of haircutting and styling. Although it is impossible to cover everything you will need to know in one book, we hope that we have given you the need-to-know information to get you started or to further your career as a barber or stylist serving the needs of the growing number of men looking for haircutting and styling services. We wish you the best of luck!

INDEX

NOTES